JORDEN BEACON

The Science of Longevity and Sleep

Insights on Aging, Health, and Living Better

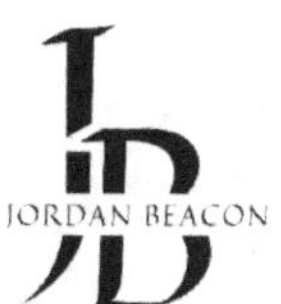

Contents

I

Understanding Longevity

1

Introduction to Longevity

People have long sought a guide to longevity. Longevity does not have to be understood as life span. There are many ways to improve the quality of life and how to work on the development and deepening of health effectively. To think about the quality of life, so that one does not survive and is still active, many body and mind styles teach. It teaches the unity of body and mind.

You can find interesting information in the statistics of the age structure of the world population. People in China, Tibet, Japan, and India live to the age of one hundred and twenty years. They are cultures with a tradition of natural health care. A country where the cult of nature and its power and energy has been cultivated and honored since ancient times. That closeness to nature, often missing nowadays, provided the basis for health and longevity. The scientific discipline that deals with the question and issue of longevity is called "anti-aging" - the science of maintaining and extending age. But it is often forgotten that taking care only of the physical area is not enough. It is very important to keep your brain active, to be able to breathe and manage your emotions. Health and healthy living are good vehicles for marketing activities.

Both women and men hear more and more about health and long life, beauty, physical freshness, and attractiveness.

Old age and aging have become a kind of phenomenon today. The number of aging people is increasing and due to this, there is more discussion about old age, aging, and longevity. In the Czech Republic, but also the surrounding European countries, there is an increase in long-lived people, i.e. people who live to be 90 years old or more.

Aging, thanks to advances in medicine and other changed circumstances, has become an expected and experienced phase of life for most people (Leissmann, 2010). Old age is the final stage of the aging process and perhaps that is why it is discussed more often in our society. There is an increase in the number of aging people who are dependent not only on the help of their closest relatives but also on the help of the entire society (Koubská, 2011). Most of us would like to live to a healthy and comfortable old age, to have family around us, and to live to a healthy old age (Liessmann, 2010). After all, old age can be pleasant and doesn't always have to bother us.

Phasing of human age

In most countries, the phasing of the human age according to the proposal of the World Health Organization (WHO) is accepted.

- 60 - 74 years - early old age
- 75 – 89 years old – own age
- 90 - and more - longevity

Other divisions of age

- 65 – 74 – young seniors
- 75 – 84 – old seniors
- 85 years and over – very old seniors

This division respects the demographic development in recent years. The population structure of society in all developed countries has changed. This structure has changed in terms of increasing life expectancy. This is an indication of the age we are likely to live to from birth.

From a Nursing Point of View

The physician recommends distinguishing the following categories of seniors):

Fit – regardless of their age, seniors maintain very good fitness, perform physically demanding activities, and manage even more demanding medical procedures, post-operative rehabilitation of the musculoskeletal system is fast for them. Seniors require minimal modifications to nursing procedures.

Independent - seniors manage activities of daily living (ADLs) well and under normal circumstances do not need any major support from family members, their surroundings, or care services (they manage household management and shopping, etc.). However, these people fail in situations where they impose an unusual burden (febrile illnesses, post-operative conditions, the necessity of walking up stairs, etc.). In the home environment, they require intervention in the event of an extraordinary load, during hospitalization they usually do not require special measures.

Fragile (frail) – seniors, are at risk of sudden decompensation of their health status (e.g. recurrent heart failure) or functional status (falls), they cannot cope with stressful situations (e.g. the development of a delirious state when the environment changes), they need permanent help with more demanding activities of daily life (the so-called instrumental ADL or IADL – e.g. shopping, cooking, household management). In the home environment, they require a nursing dispensary with interventions, often monitoring using emergency care systems (emergency calls), in institutional care, increased supervision is needed to prevent immobilization syndrome or delirious states, upon discharge to the home environment, usually the activation of field services (nursing service) or instruction families.

Dependent – seniors are unable to manage even ordinary self-care, they require help with eating, hygiene, dressing, using the toilet, and moving from bed.

Completely dependent – seniors are long-term or permanently confined to bed due to a quantitative or qualitative disorder of consciousness, therefore they require active provision of an anti-decubitus regimen, hydration, and nutrition. They are at risk of developing immobilization syndrome

The Aging Process

Aging affects the entire population. Aging is a long-term process that is influenced by two factors. Genetic factors are given to a person from birth and factors from the surrounding world. The interaction of both factors creates the uniqueness and peculiarity of how an individual will go through the aging process quickly or slowly. Aging and old people have only several years in common. Everyone ages differently, at a different pace. In some periods we age faster, in others more slowly. But watch out! Chronologically speaking, we all age the same. The calendar age can therefore be understood as the only value according to which we can compare age groups from different countries of the world with each other.

Longevity

According to the World Health Organization, people older than 90 are considered long-lived in our country. Various studies show that if a person lived in a healthy environment and was not killed by certain malignant or chronic diseases, he could live to be a hundred years old or more.

1. Long-lived people naturally enjoy regular exercise (walking, gardening, activities they do more for fun than as a health obligation).
2. Their personality is balanced but lively, they have a zest for life but don't show excessive emotions that lead to outbursts of anger or moments of panic.
3. They avoid nostalgia, they don't live in the past. That would mean thinking about the times when they were even younger, faster, and stronger, and that can be daunting. Instead, they live in the present and are excited about today's activities.
4. They are successful in what they do, even if they set modest goals, when they achieve them, they see for themselves that it extends their lives. They are more proud of their work than themselves.
5. They are moderate in their habits, eat a varied diet without fads, regularly consume a daily combination of meat and vegetables, and also drink moderate amounts of alcohol.
6. Their way of life is like a daily routine without confusion and

stress.

7. Their eyes shine, and their sense of humor does not leave them even in old age.

The countries with the oldest population in Europe (median age) in 2011 were Germany (44.6 years), Italy (43.5 years), Finland (42.1 years), Greece (42.1 years), and Austria (42,0 years). Ireland (34.7 years), Iceland (35.0 years), and Macedonia (36.1 years) have the youngest populations; in the Czech Republic in 2011 the median age was 39.6 years. The population in Europe aged the most from 2002 to 2011 in Liechtenstein (by 4.3 years), in Germany (by 4 years), in Lithuania (by 3.5 years), in Greece (by 3.3 years) and equally by 3.2 years in Austria, the Netherlands and Macedonia. The population is aging the least in Sweden (by 1.2 years), in Hungary and Estonia (by 1.4 years), and in Bulgaria (by 1.5 years); in the Czech Republic by 1.7 years."

The phenomenon of population aging is becoming the most urgent problem in developed European countries, and population aging has a significant impact on the entire society. More and more funds need to be spent on health care and the social system. Quality and good aging do not only depend on the social structure, it also on individual actions and attitudes toward the elderly. The quality of life of the long-lived must be as good as possible. However, it is necessary to think about this already in youth.

Exploring the Factors that Cause Aging

Aging is the sum of all the mechanisms that change the functions of a living being, interfere with the maintenance of physiological balance, and ultimately lead to death. The aging process is a complex, gradual process, depending on many biological factors. Scientists have always shown a special interest in aging and the search for approaches to studying this phenomenon.

Research has shown that aging is controlled by genetic factors and biological processes inherent to humanity.

To slow down this natural process and increase life expectancy, the first step is to understand the causes of aging: how it affects living organisms, and what factors influence life expectancy.

There are 7 main causes: genomic damage, epigenetic factors, telomere shortening, unfolded protein response, mitochondrial dysfunction, cellular aging, and stem cell depletion.

DNA repair errors

The genome is the sum of the genetic information of an individual or species. The genome is a map for building the entire organism. Genetic information is mainly stored in the cell nucleus in the form of DNA molecules. A section of DNA that specifies the sequence of a specific polypeptide or functional RNA represents a gene. The human genome contains between 25,000 and 30,000 genes.

However, DNA molecules do not lie free in the cell nucleus; they are packaged together with histone proteins in chromosomes. Chromosomes contain all genetic information and are replicated with each cell division.

Throughout life, cells divide many times, resulting in genetic material constantly being reproduced in living systems and passed on to newly created daughter cells. During cell division, genetic errors that are formed during DNA replication are quite common. These are called DNA replication errors. Replication errors lead to disruption of cell function and can affect remaining tissue if the cell is not eliminated by triggering apoptosis (cell death) or senescence (deterioration of cell function).

The body also has a system that repairs DNA molecules modified during replication. The system uses proteins and enzymes. PARP1 is involved in DNA and sirtuin repair, as well as in the regulation of gene expression, chromatin remodeling, and mitochondrial function. NAD+ is a cosubstrate of PARP. With age, the expression of PARP proteins increases, which indicates frequent replication errors and the need to eliminate them. In response to DNA damage due to PARP, the cell also very quickly depletes NAD+ reserves, which leads to cell death.

Activation of the PARP enzyme can induce overexpression of P53 protein. The P53 protein represents another cell life cycle control system. P53 is responsible for the elimination of carcinogenic cells and helps prolong the life of organs, preventing the development of cancer cells. However, the more the protein is activated, the more it accelerates the aging process, leading to increased cell destruction and loss of tissue homogeneity.

Mechanism of telomeric repeat shortening

The ability of diploid cells to proliferate is limited. This process is regulated by telomeres. Telomeres have a protective effect on DNA. Telomeres are the part of the chromosome that does not contain genetic information and are destroyed throughout life with each replication until they completely disappear. Because the DNA is no longer protected, important information is chewed up during replication, leading to cell apoptosis or the creation of a cancer cell. The enzyme telomerase ensures complete replication of telomeres. It is found only in stem, embryonic, and cancer cells. The presence of this enzyme in cancer cells explains why they are immortal: they can divide endlessly without stopping their "biological clock." The work of this enzyme is of great scientific interest, however, its activation may be associated with the induction of malignant transformation.

Telomere shortening can be compared to a biological clock, which activates cell aging as soon as time runs out. This mechanism limits the lifespan of all cells and is therefore central.

Epigenetic mechanisms and aging

Epigenetics is the study of the mechanisms that control genome expression. Gene expression can vary depending on environmental factors. Organs exhibit this variability: each cell has similar genetic information but different functions, showing differences in gene expression depending on the environment.

There are several epigenetic mechanisms for regulating gene activity:

Methylation reactions

Methylation is an epigenetic modification of the genome through the addition or removal of a methyl group. Methylation reactions can activate, inhibit gene expression, or increase the likelihood of mutation. The methylation process affects estrogen receptors, tumor suppressors, and other important genes. Epigenetic modifications associated with methylation increase with age and can lead to serious health problems.

Chromatin remodeling

In the nucleus, DNA takes the form of chromatin, which allows the genetic material to be compacted. With age, chromatin remodeling decreases and chromosome stability decreases, which is accompanied by premature aging.

Histone modification

Histones are proteins around which DNA is wrapped. They make up the majority of the chromosome. Any modification of histone components can alter gene expression. For example, some hormones are responsible for the addition or removal of histone components (sirtuins, NF-kB) and influence genome stability. Histone modification influences lifespan through modifications in the expression of certain genes.

Disturbance of protein conformation as a cause of aging

Proteins are represented by a polypeptide chain consisting of a sequence of amino acids. Proteins work due to their conformational structure: secondary, tertiary, and quaternary. Protein folding represents the physical process of folding by which a protein becomes functionally active.

Studies have shown that disruption of the protein folding process forms the pathophysiological basis of many age-related diseases of various etiologies, including Alzheimer's disease, Parkinson's disease, and others.

The consequences of disruption of conformational structures are associated with the accumulation of protein aggregates of incorrect conformation.

Mitochondrial dysfunction and age

Mitochondria are cellular organelles responsible for maintaining cellular respiration and the synthesis of ATP, the main source of energy. Mitochondria have their DNA, called mtDNA.

Mitochondrial dysfunction is a major cause of aging due to the vital role of mitochondria in cells. Age-related dysfunction occurs with age and can lead to cell death. Its cause is oxidative stress, a violation of the cell-mitochondrial connection.

Cellular aging

Cellular senescence occurs when a cell's age increases and its function decreases. The cell stops dividing and changes its activity. Senescent cells can be seen at all stages of life. With age, their number increases in some tissues, causing their heterogeneity.

The mechanism of cellular aging is beneficial in youth. It protects the body from the proliferation of cancer cells but requires an effective immune system to eliminate senescent cells. As we age, the effectiveness of the immune system decreases, and stem cell renewal occurs less frequently.

Stem cells

Stem cells are undifferentiated cells that do not belong to any specific organ and can therefore generate specialized cells through "cellular differentiation."

Stem cells make it possible to renew cells in an organ; they are stored in the body and used when necessary.

Some cells age and die regularly and require replacement. The lifespan of an erythrocyte is on average 120 days. Other organs may grow and require more tissue (for example, the uterus during pregnancy). Some organs do not have stem cells and therefore cannot be renewed when damaged, for example, the heart, or pancreas.

With aging, tissues also do not recover due to slower cell division and lack of replacement of stem cells. This is due to overexpression of cell cycle-blocking proteins or accumulation of DNA damage on stem cells.

Stem cell depletion is one of the main causes of aging, as it prevents cell renewal and causes organ aging. Understanding how stem cells work will be vital for regenerative medicine in the future.

The above reasons are potentially responsible for changes in body functions. Some of these underlie beneficial mechanisms that become deleterious with age, as is the case with cellular senescence and the DNA repair system. The mechanisms prevent the development of cancer, but as their activity becomes too high, they fail and degeneration of the body accelerates.

Other causes are simple mechanisms that develop slowly over time (mitochondrial dysfunction, telomere shortening). It is necessary to understand them if we ever want to work on them to potentially slow down aging and increase human lifespan.

2

Nutrition for Longevity

Our daily eating habits, which seem to have no immediate impact on our well-being, have a systemic impact on our health, experts emphasize. Poor nutrition increases the risk of cardiovascular diseases, arterial hypertension, obesity, diabetes, and cancer. What rules should you follow at the table to avoid dangerous diseases and maintain health for many years?

The Role of Nutrition in Longevity

The Menu Changes with the Person

At the level of intuition and common sense, it is clear that nutrition should be commensurate with how much energy a person spends: you cannot eat a lot during sedentary work and, conversely, go hungry during heavy workloads. If you focus on the numbers, then 2000 kilocalories per day are enough for the average person, clarifies the chief freelance specialist of the Russian Ministry of Health for preventive medicine, Sergei Boytsov:

For example, during a period of rapid growth, a 15-to 16-year-old teenage boy can eat a large amount of food: it is easily digested and does not leave any unpleasant consequences in the form of fat deposits. But already at the age of 18-20, nutrition should become more moderate. Otherwise, by the age of 25, a man may develop visceral (internal) fat deposits in the abdominal cavity, omentum, mesentery, and liver, in other words, a small tummy will appear, and by 35-40 abdominal obesity will appear (excess fat in the upper half of the body and on the abdomen), and the risk of cardiovascular disease will increase. Unfortunately, this is what the stereotypical portrait of a Russian looks like today. At the age of 30-60 years, our men, on average, consume 3500-4000 Kk. To balance their diet, they can safely cut the amount of food in half.

The "secret of the pyramid" will help an adult to adhere to the correct diet. The daily set of products should follow a simple scheme: the basis of the "food pyramid" is vegetables and fruits (for example, for 1 day, one serving of vegetable salad and at least two large fruits are enough, the simplest option is two apples).

In second place are cereals (morning porridge, grain bread).

Next - legumes (peas and legumes contain large amounts of vegetable protein, i.e. essential amino acids).

As for fish and meat, nutritionists recommend choosing fish from cold seas and eating it at least twice a week; It is enough to eat meat 1-2 times a week. At the same time, focus on the turkey, rabbit, skinless chicken (it contains a lot of fatty acids, fats, and cholesterol), and lean varieties of beef.

Set an alarm for lunch

A person should have 3 meals and 2 snacks daily, experts say. Moreover, meals do not mean desserts and snacks, but full meals - breakfast, lunch, dinner (porridge, soups, meat, chicken, vegetables, fruits). You should have dinner at least two hours before bedtime. The main products for snacks are fruits and vegetables, for sweets - dried fruits, candied fruits, fruit chips.

Put a lock on the sweet life

The daily menu should contain as little sugar and sweets as possible. According to the recommendations of the World Health Organization (WHO), the daily sugar intake for a healthy person should not exceed 50 grams (about 10 teaspoons). In case of presence or predisposition to chronic diseases - for example, obesity, hypertension, carbohydrate metabolism disorders, this amount is reduced to 30 grams, and in case of kidney disease, diabetes mellitus - to 15-20 grams.

Today, sugar is used mainly as a flavor enhancer; the "sugar boom" began in the mid-20th century, and it is with excess consumption of sugar and sugar-containing products that scientists associate a surge in obesity, type 2 diabetes, and cardiovascular diseases in developed countries. A diet saturated with sugar negatively changes metabolism and provokes the accelerated formation of atherosclerotic plaques. Also, excessive sugar consumption contributes to the accumulation of excess intracellular fluid in tissues and swelling.

The situation is aggravated by the fact that we not only add sugar to our dishes and drinks but also consume so-called "added sugar" in store-bought products. Even mustard, mayonnaise, and ketchup contain sugar, not to mention sweet drinks, juices, syrups, soda, milk chocolate, flour, and confectionery products. This additional sugar essentially has no nutritional value, only increasing the energy value of the dish. "Hidden" sugar must be taken into account when calculating the daily norm.

How to do it? According to Russian law, manufacturers are required to indicate on the label the amount of sugar in the product. For example, yogurts with various fruit additives, even with low-fat content, contain approximately 10 grams of sugar, in total 3 cups of yogurt per day is already 30 grams of sugar. A tablespoon of honey contains one-third of your daily sugar intake.

Remove the salt shaker from the table

It is important to consume less salt in its pure form and minimize excessively salty foods (hard cheeses, sausages, pickles, herring, smoked meats, canned food, mayonnaise, ketchup, soy sauce), experts advise. As with sugar, WHO limits the daily salt intake for a healthy person to no more than 7 g per day (one tablespoon). If there is a risk or presence of chronic diseases - 4 - 5 g.

"Salt restriction is one of the main factors in the prevention of arterial hypertension, and low-salt diets have an excellent antihypertensive effect!" - assures the chief freelance nutritionist of the Department of Health of the Tyumen Region, Elena Dorodneva.

Salt retains fluid, so when you consume too much salt, fluid accumulates in the body. And this is the reason for the increase in diastolic ("lower") blood pressure at a young age. Also, a person becomes insensitive to many medications - so-called resistance occurs. In addition, "looseness" and lethargy appear. The face swells, especially the eyelids, and in the evenings the legs swell.

"According to epidemiological studies of the Federal Statistics Service from 2012, approximately 60% of the adult population exceed the permissible salt standards by almost 2 times - they consume 11 g of salt per day. And these statistics do not take into account additional salting, which is one of the main mechanisms of excess salt consumption," notes Sergei Boytsov, chief freelance specialist of the Russian Ministry of Health for preventive medicine.

To control salt consumption, experts recommend not adding additional salt after preparing a dish at the table. Use more spices - various mixtures of herbs and sea salt, pepper, sea, rock, iodized salt (5-6 g of iodized salt per day is a good prevention of iodine deficiency). Treat pickles, smoked meats, canned food, and hard cheeses as snacks - eat 1 - 2 pieces.

Put a bold cross on a bold one

The fifth rule is less fat. It is advisable to reduce or abandon fatty meat products (chicken, turkey, rabbit, and lean beef are allowed), fatty dairy products (yogurt no more than 5%, sour cream no more than 10%), products with a high content of trans-fatty acids (almost all confectionery products: cakes, sweets, waffles, chips and everything that crunches).

"Today we spend much less energy than our ancestors to eat fatty foods in huge quantities," explains Elena Dorodneva. "To eat 20% sour cream and whole dairy products, you need to live in the early 20th century - walk, do not use the elevator, do not work on the ground, and engage in physical labor!"

Simple Tips for Healthy Aging

Keep moving

When your body starts to protest against certain activities, it's easy to sit back and relax. However, this will not make you feel better, say health professionals. "Stay active, walk a lot, train the muscles if necessary, and pay extra attention to balance,". The advice is:

1. Exercise at least 2.5 hours per week. This doesn't have to be complicated: a walk with a friend also counts! The most important thing is that you don't sit still.
2. Do exercises that strengthen your muscles and bones at least twice a week. For example, you can participate in Nederland in Beweging or search for free videos with exercises and exercise activities on YouTube.

Eat enough protein

Professor Lisette de Groot from Wageningen University conducts research into the nutrition of older people. It is a given that your muscle strength and muscle mass decrease as you get older. Professor De Groot and her team are investigating how you can stop or even reverse this process. A combination of strength training and protein-rich nutrition appears to increase muscle mass and strength in the elderly, according to their research.

You will find free protein-rich recipes on the Nutrition Center website.

Challenge your brain

Many people over the age of 65 are afraid of losing their memory or developing a form of dementia. And while it's true that some connections in your brain weaken or disappear after a few decades, that doesn't mean you can't do anything about it! The Brain Foundation mentions 3 things you can do yourself to keep your brain healthy:

- Healthy food
- Enough sleep
- Exercise regularly

In addition, it is important to keep challenging your brain. In her book 'The 50+ Brain', neuropsychologist Margriet Sitskoorn describes how you can keep your brain healthy by doing new things. "By challenging yourself cognitively, the brain will create more connections," she tells Nemo Kennislink. "It doesn't have to be something completely new. If you like modern art and are now going to make bobbin lace, that's okay. Older people often think they have to do Sudoku; you should only do that if you like it. What matters is that you challenge yourself a little." For example, another professor of Neuropsychology, Erik Scherder, describes that he started playing the violin after the age of 65. Quite a challenge, but it makes him fitter and happier.

3

Sleep, Stress, and Longevity

Importance of Sleep in Longevity

Good sleep is an integral part of a healthy lifestyle. However, in the modern world, more and more people are faced with sleep problems, which negatively affect their physical and psychological well-being. In this chapter, we'll look at the key aspects of healthy sleep and present effective approaches to help you achieve physical well-being and mental balance.

To get the most benefit from your sleep, it is important to monitor its quality and duration. It is recommended to sleep at least 7-8 hours a day and create comfortable conditions for this.

Let's take a closer look at the main aspects of life that are affected by healthy sleep and understand how to get the maximum benefit from it for our body.

Sleep improves physical well-being

Quality sleep plays a key role in regulating metabolism and hormone levels in the body.

Lack of sleep can lead to metabolic disorders and increased levels of the hormone ghrelin, which increases appetite and promotes the accumulation of fat in the body.

Lack of sleep can also increase levels of cortisol, a hormone that is involved in regulating stress but, when in excess, can lead to obesity and other diseases.

During sleep, other important hormones are also produced, for example, melatonin and somatotropin, they are involved in the regulation of metabolism and general hormonal levels.

During sleep, the body restores energy, repairs damaged cells and tissues, and improves immunity.

Healthy sleep allows you to achieve full recovery after physical activity and improves the overall performance of the body.

This is especially important for athletes and people with an active lifestyle. When we sleep, our body increases its immunity to successfully fight diseases.

Growth hormone, or somatotropin, is produced during sleep and is one of the key factors influencing the body's recovery after physical activity. It speeds up recovery processes helps athletes achieve better results and prevents injuries.

Sleep stabilizes the psyche

Healthy sleep has a direct impact on memory, concentration and decision-making processes.

During sleep, information received during the day is processed. Lack of sleep can lead to poor memory, difficulty concentrating, and decreased mental productivity.

Research shows that people who get enough sleep remember information better and have sharper attention and concentration than those who get little sleep.

Sleep also helps speed up the brain's processing of information, which can make thinking more efficient. Lack of sleep, on the other hand, can lead to difficulties in making decisions and completing tasks.

Good sleep plays an important role in maintaining emotional balance and reducing stress, anxiety and depression.

During sleep, psychological resources are restored and stress levels are reduced. Good sleep helps reduce levels of stress hormones such as cortisol, which can be linked to low mood, anxiety, and depression.

Lack of sleep can lead to increased irritability, poor mood, and poor health. Research shows that people who get enough sleep have a more positive mood, feel more energetic, and are less likely to experience depression and anxiety.

Good sleep also helps improve performance and increase confidence in your abilities. People who get enough sleep are more likely to feel more emotionally stable and able to work effectively.

How to arrange the perfect sleeping place

The optimal choice of mattress, pillows, bed linen and a pleasant atmosphere play an important role in ensuring quality sleep.

Here are some recommendations for arranging the ideal sleeping place:

Mattress: select a mattress, which suits your body and the way you sleep. There are several types of mattresses including spring, springless, with shape memory. Before you make your choice, determine your individual needs, such as stiffness, support, and spring availability. Also, make sure the mattress is suitable for your size. beds. More details about choosing a mattress.

Pillow: choosepillow, which suits your sleep style. For example, for those who love to sleep on their stomachs, thinner pillows are recommended so as not to create unnecessary pressure on the neck. And to those sleeping on the side, Taller pillows may be appropriate to support the neck in the correct position. There are also special orthopedic pillows, which help you sleep comfortably, despite problems with the spine. More details about choosing a pillow.

Bed linen: selectbed sheets, which is suitable for your temperature and skin preference. Some people prefer cooler bedding, while others prefer warmer bedding. Also make sure that the bedding is a good fit for the size of your bed and is easy to wash.

Lighting: Create a comfortable sleeping environment by making sure your bedroom has the right lighting lighting. Avoid bright lights before bed and use dark curtains or sleep masks to create darkness.

Ambiance: Create a pleasant environment in your bedroom to help you relax before bed. For example, you can use scented candles or essential oil diffusers to fill your room with a pleasant aroma. Also, make sure the room temperature is comfortable - not too hot or cold.

How to improve your sleep quality?

Maintain a routine. Try to go to bed and wake up at the same time every day to get your body used to a regular schedule.

Create a calm atmosphere. Before bed, try to reduce the light and noise levels in your bedroom to create a calm atmosphere. It is also recommended to use a comfortable and soft bed, as well as good ventilation in the bedroom.

Avoid alcohol and drugs. Alcohol and drugs can negatively affect the quality of sleep and lead to insomnia.

Reduce your caffeine intake. Caffeine, found in drinks such as coffee, tea, soda, and chocolate, can interfere with sleep and cause awakenings at night.

Get physically active. Regular physical activity can help improve your sleep quality. However, try not to exercise immediately before bed to avoid stimulating your body.

Avoid eating before bed. It is not recommended to consume heavy foods, alcohol, or caffeine before bed, as this can make it difficult to fall asleep.

Use relaxation techniques. Relaxation techniques such as meditation, yoga, deep breathing, and progressive muscle relaxation can help reduce stress and promote sleep.

Avoid using gadgets before bed. Using gadgets such as smartphones, tablets, and computers before bed can make it difficult to fall asleep. It is better to read a book or listen to calm music.

These tips can help improve your sleep quality and combat mild insomnia. However, if you have serious sleep disorders, it is best to consult a doctor to get professional help and appropriate treatment.

How does stress management help prevent disease?

Stress is a normal reaction of the body to any irritants. This reaction evolutionarily helps a person cope with difficulties and contributes to the development of adaptation. That is, thanks to the reaction to stress, humans have survived as a species. But if stress is excessive and prolonged, it can harm your health.

What kind of stress is there?

The scientist Hans Selye, almost 100 years ago, highlighted:

1. Eustress is a useful, mobilizing stress, overcoming which a person feels satisfied.
2. Distress is excessive, chronic stress that is destructive and leads to exhaustion. It is not only accompanied by negative emotions but also causes several adverse effects at the physiological level and can cause illness.

The number of stress factors is of great importance. Low doses of stress factors have a positive stimulating effect on the body (hormesis), and high doses lead to a breakdown of protective mechanisms.

How does stress manifest itself physiologically and psychologically?

The stress response occurs in response to demands placed on the body and does not depend on the nature of the stressors. Accordingly, stress arises from stressors of various types associated with potential threats. The body's response to stress activates the hypothalamic-pituitary-adrenal axis and, as a result, the release of cortisol. Under the influence of stress, the psychological state also changes. A state of excitement and hypermobilization occurs.

You are late for an important meeting because you are stuck in traffic. You feel irritated, angry, indignant. The pulse may become faster and the muscles will tense up. There is nothing you can do to change the situation, but the body perceives warning signs and prepares for "fight or flight." This is an example of the relationship between physiology and psychology.

Psychological stress (the emotions you experience, for example, when stuck in a traffic jam) provokes physiological stress and changes in your body. But it happens the other way around, when a problem in the body, for example, pain, causes a psycho-emotional response.

What does science say about the connection between stress and disease?

Today there is quite a lot of research on the connection between stress and the development of somatic and mental disorders. The connection between stress and mental illness is stronger than the connection with physical illness. The risk of developing a mental disorder increases 2-7 times within 6 months of a stressful event (Paykel ES).

The INTERHEART study (2004) found that people with myocardial infarction reported higher rates of work and home stress, financial-related stress, and major life events in the past year. Since IHD and heart attack are directly related to hypertension, it is worth noting that "stress hormones" cause an increase in blood pressure, therefore arterial hypertension is a stress-related disease.

A stress reaction can be one of the causes of stomach and duodenal ulcers, and can also affect the development of type 2 diabetes. The most demonstrative is the occurrence of diabetes after prolonged experiences and acute shock, emotionally significant situations. A classic example of diabetes mellitus that occurs after emotional upheaval is the diabetes of stockbrokers after a fall in prices on the Chicago Stock Exchange.

Several studies have shown that chronic stress has an overall suppressive effect on the immune response, reducing the body's ability to initiate a rapid and effective immune response (Salleh MR)

However, in a study by T. L. Lindquist et al. It has been shown that the risk of developing certain somatic disorders in people of working age is associated not so much with the level of stress but with the characteristics of the strategies used to overcome it, as well as with lifestyle characteristics.

What types of stress exist?

In everyday life, we encounter social, cognitive, or physiological stressors in various situations. According to this point of view, there are two different types of stressors:

1. Physiological stress manifests itself as unpleasant sensory, subjective experiences associated with potential tissue damage and bodily threats. Physical stress can also include various bodily conditions, for example, pain, hunger, and hypothermia.
2. Psychosocial stress is triggered by situations of social threat, including social evaluation, rejection, and achievement situations that require achieving a set goal.

What can be a source of stress?

The need to be connected to other people and to maintain a social self are basic psychological needs. If the satisfaction of these needs is threatened, for example, as a result of negative evaluation of the activity by other people, then social threat and, consequently, stress arises.

Social evaluation as well as cognitive achievements with unpredictable outcomes cause an increased cortisol response, which is accompanied by subjective reports of stress and negative experiences. People with increased sensitivity to social evaluation also have an increased cortisol response to acute stressors such as achievement tasks or social exclusion.

In general, various events in life can be sources of stress; this largely depends on the prism through which a person views the world and which is formed from the characteristics of upbringing, culture, mentality, and life experience.

How to manage stress?

In today's world, everyone needs to know about stress management. What methods and techniques help you survive and manage stress?

Physical activity, in addition to its basic necessity for physical and mental health, can be used at a time when there is a feeling of extreme anxiety or tension. For example, jogging, a couple of dozen intense squats, or push-ups will help neutralize stress hormones at a physiological level.

Breathing techniques have a certain effect (and the exhalation should be longer than the inhalation) or square breathing when in addition to inhaling for 4 counts, you need to hold your breath, then exhale, and then hold it again before the next inhalation (all for an equal number of counts). By thus provoking a slight oxygen deficiency, we trigger the mechanism of "saving strength" in the body, and it stops being spent on mobilization.

The most proven ways to cope with stress are techniques from cognitive behavioral therapy and its types. Emotional regulation and mindfulness techniques, as well as various other interventions aimed at reducing anxiety levels and developing a tolerance for this experience, are in no way suppressive. That is, the task of the exercises and techniques is to ensure that the feeling of anxiety does not seem unbearable, but does not "paralyze" it. Various planning and decision-making techniques can be used.

The reaction of our muscles to stress is associated with biologically active substances released in our body during that same stress. And the analyst W. Reich wrote about the "muscle shell" of the Austrians back in the first half of the last century. When stressed, muscle tension can occur, which, of course, is also important to work with. Various mindfulness techniques aimed at bodily sensations (for example, a body scanner), muscle relaxation techniques, yoga, and massage are suitable here.

How can a healthy lifestyle help prevent stress-related illnesses?

To increase stress resistance and reduce the risks of developing various anxiety and mood disorders due to stress, it is essential to maintain physical health. This is based on:

1. nutritious food rich in all nutrients
2. healthy sleep (try to fall asleep and wake up at the same time, following a routine, and sleep for at least 7 hours)
3. physical activity (from 150 to 300 minutes per week according to WHO recommendations)
4. regular medical examinations to prevent chronic diseases and take care of your physical health
5. limiting or giving up alcohol and other bad habits
6. compliance with the work and rest regime. In a series of tasks and workloads, he often remains unattended. But overexertion, which is already stress associated with the amount of work or working conditions (for example, when it is difficult to influence the result and it is impossible to feel one's the importance of professional competence), has a strong impact on our ability to cope with other stresses

Psychologists and doctors recommend no more than 40 working hours a week; more is no longer physiological. In addition, each person has his threshold, and it is also important to remember and listen to yourself:

1. Take breaks during the workday
2. Learn to "slow down" and pay attention to what is happening around you
3. Try simple meditation techniques

4

Strategies for Aging Well

The process of population aging occurs in conditions of a simultaneous decline in the birth rate, and the mortality rate is also high. In connection with the increase in the number of older people in the socio-demographic structure of the population of the Russian Federation, research in the field of life activity of older people, understanding their place and role in society is becoming relevant. Institutions for social protection of the population are developing new forms and methods for improving the quality of social services for older citizens, taking into account current problems of their life.

It is difficult to unambiguously characterize this life period, either on the positive or negative side. Some scientists consider it as a set of losses or losses - economic, social, individual, which can negatively affect the future life of an elderly person. On the other hand, it is at this age that a person analyzes his life path, sees what he has achieved, and has a desire to share experiences and give advice. You can find a large number of positive aspects in your new social status.

In society, there are a large number of social stereotypes regarding older people that influence the choice of aging strategy, which can be understood as the method, pace and lifestyle chosen by a person after retirement. Social stereotypes and patterns affect a person's subjective relationship not only to society, but also to himself; they influence the self-perception of older people.

Considering the modern family and the system of intergenerational relationships, D. Bromley notes that the traditional patriarchal family is disintegrating, that old men - fathers of the family no longer play their former role, that the younger generation does not need the support of the old, and the old are moving away from the family altogether, not playing the role of grandfathers and grandmothers.

In addition, there are trends towards a progressive increase in loneliness in old age and old age at present and in the future. Many elderly people have to face such a problem as changing their living space, which is an additional difficulty in old age and greatly affects the mood of the elderly person. Old people end up in boarding homes for various reasons.

Basically, people living in a boarding house have problems in relation-ships with relatives, sometimes they lose contact with their family, the latter is most often the reason for ending up in a boarding school, which greatly affects the emotional state of a person. He has to put in a lot more effort when adapting to new living conditions. The nature of adaptation is greatly influenced by the life attitude of the elderly person, his character, and ability to cope with difficulties. The more optimistic the mood, the more effective the aging strategy is.

Today, it is important to change the course of life in an aging society.

It is especially important to include older people living in a boarding house in the active life. Unlike a family, living in a residential facility is a completely different way of life.

Criteria for choosing an aging strategy

Effective aging strategy (constructive)	Ineffective aging strategy (not constructive)
High/medium level of readiness for age-related changes (attitude towards one's own old age)High/medium level of readiness for age-related changes (attitude towards one's own old age)	Low level of readiness for age-related changes (attitude towards one's own old age)
Maintaining an active lifestyle in old age	Preference for a passive life position in old age
Maintaining constant (regular/periodic) communication with family	Irregularity/lack of communication with family
Positive contacts with your immediate environment	Negative contacts with the immediate environment (aggression)

Criteria for choosing an aging Strategy

In addition, when determining the aging strategy, observation methods and interviews with an institution specialist were used. The results obtained were tabulated for three components "Social activity", which included indicators of the frequency of attending events and the way of spending free time, passive/active; component - "Relationships with others", which reveals the nature of communication, the degree of sociability with neighbors living in the institution; in the content of the "Social situation" component, the main thing is the reason for ending up in a boarding school and the presence of contact with relatives, the frequency of communication with them. Based on the results of filling out the tables, a conclusion was made about the effectiveness/ineffectiveness of the chosen aging strategy. The results showed that out of 30 people surveyed, 16 had an effective aging strategy, of which 6 were men and 10 were women.

An ineffective aging strategy occurs in 14 people, of which 7 are men and 7 are women. The predominance of an effective aging strategy can be explained by the predominance of active leisure, vigorous activity, and hobbies among women. Men find themselves communicating with their neighbors, but they are less likely to take part in the leisure life of the boarding house. Since the cognitive level of readiness for age-related changes in women is at a higher level than in men, they adapt better to the characteristics of age. This is more difficult for men. Relationships with family play an important role in choosing the effectiveness of an aging strategy. It should be noted that women keep in touch more regularly than men.

Every elderly person wants to feel needed and involved in something important and relevant to others. In an old person, according to V. Henry, the motivation for work changes. An elderly person strives to work, but no longer to support himself, but for the sake of work, which acquires an emotional overtones. The old man analyzes his work only about himself, and not to social activities, as the ability to do the work, as self-esteem.

At first glance, it may seem that there are not many opportunities in a residential care facility to fully realize the potential of an elderly person. A boarding home is stereotypically perceived as an institution where old people go to live out their lives. However in fact, with the help of ordinary things you can create a completely special atmosphere for living. For example, if calm classical music is played unobtrusively in the lobby of an institution, this will help create a more pleasant atmosphere of life in general.

When creating conditions, it is necessary to take into account that people at this age begin to especially value some traditions that are associated with their youth. Tradition generally has its special role in each team, which unites people. It's good if such a tradition is created in the institution. Not just to celebrate holidays together, but to come up with something that will unite people for such joint activities that will be interesting to everyone. Considering that people of different ages with different interests live in a boarding school, you can simply help people organize into clubs. Someone, having retired, starts knitting, and someone has free time to cook. By getting together, older people can feel included, and useful, and even learn something new.

In residential institutions, various forms of organizing the free time of the elderly are practiced, such as artistic, applied, and creative activities; holidays, competitions, checkers tournaments, excursions, and games. The more residents of the boarding school are involved in active leisure, the better their emotional state. In addition to active recreation, do not forget about simple pastimes: reading, watching TV, listening to the radio.

In addition, today there are many methods known that can help residents of an inpatient facility feel needed, interesting interlocutors, reveal hidden potential, and increase interest in life. An example is the biographical method, which is considered quite effective for motivating the life activity of people who have entered the late period of adulthood. Using this method, an elderly person gets the opportunity to share his life experience, talk about the peculiarities of his destiny, and at the same time understand how his past influenced the formation of his present. The process of remembering itself, even without its in-depth psychological analysis, can have a very strong psychotherapeutic effect and contribute to the emergence of a positive self-perception. It is advisable to practice in every possible way various meetings and correspondence between elderly residents of a boarding school and residents of nearby kindergartens and schools. It would help if you also referred to photographs once given as postcards, which will help the memories become brighter.

In addition, there is a method of memoir therapy, which is an effective remedy for depression, which often occurs among new residents of an institution in the process of adapting to new living conditions. This method is an offshoot of the biographical methessential important here that an elderly person tries to focus only on the positive aspects of his life. You can suggest creating a family book so that his descendants know more about the history of their family.

It is important that in a boarding home, a person does not feel like just a client of the institution. It is necessary that he can become part of the community of residents. To do this, the staff of the institution must be well aware of the characteristics of people of the third age and treat various manifestations of their character with understanding and, if necessary, correct the situation. At the center of the relationship should be a person's rich and valuable life experience, which others treat with respect.

II

How We Age

5

Understanding the Cellular Processes Involved in Aging

Normal human somatic cells have very limited division capabilities, and when they are exhausted, they enter the aging phase. It is believed that the cellular aging process is a response to extensive and irreversible DNA damage located within telomeric and/or non-telomeric sequences of the genome. The accumulation of this type of damage is caused primarily by oxidative stress, which increases due to impaired mitochondrial function. Old cells accumulate in tissues as the body ages, which is causally linked to the development of many old-age diseases, including cancer. The aim of the work, prepared exactly 50 years after Leonard Hayflick discovered the connections between cell aging and the aging of the organism as a whole, is to present the state of knowledge on the molecular determinants of aging at the cellular level, with particular emphasis on the role of oxidative stress, aging effectors in the cell cycle, and markers. this process and the impact of old cells on the development of specific age-related pathologies.

Introduction

Modern science offers many definitions of the aging process, and the selection of the appropriate one is usually dictated by the specific aspect of the life of the organism to which this process applies. Biologically, this phenomenon can be defined as a set of dynamic changes, dependent on the passage of time and environmental factors acting at the structural and functional level of the body. This definition emphasizes the universality and physiological role of this process. In the medical aspect, aging is assessed rather pejoratively, which results from the accompanying increase in the incidence of many age-related diseases, significantly deteriorating the quality and limiting the life expectancy of older people. To understand the nature of changes occurring during aging, we most often use cellular models, which constitute a kind of "microworld" reflecting the regularities that govern entire organisms. Bearing in mind that last year has passed 50 years since the exhaustion of cell division potential was first linked to the aging process of the human body as a whole, it seems worth presenting the current state of knowledge about the molecular mechanisms governing cellular aging, as well as the relationships between this phenomenon and the development of many age-related diseases, including cancer.

Cellular model of aging

Aging is a complex process and is the result of biochemical and physiological phenomena occurring at various levels of body organization, from a single cell to tissues and organs. In a unanimous opinion, the aging process, which takes place at the cellular level, is one of the best models for studying this phenomenon, which results from the possibility of in-depth insight into molecular events occurring at the level of macromolecules, as well as subjecting cells to appropriate manipulations (e.g. the influence of environmental factors, interventions genetic), allowing the identification of changes in cell metabolism that may be a direct cause or effect of the aging process.

Mechanisms of somatic cell aging

Normal human somatic cells have very limited division capabilities, and when they are exhausted, they enter the aging phase. It is believed that the cellular aging process is a response to extensive and irreversible DNA damage located within telomeric and/or non-telomeric sequences of the genome.

Phenotype of old cells

Cells that have reached the aging phase, either as a result of undergoing a critical number of divisions or under the influence of specific stressors, differ fundamentally from proliferating cells in many morphological and functional features, collectively referred to as the old cell phenotype. The most classic features of old cells include an increase in size (hypertrophy), flattening, loss of uniform shape, multinucleation, and vacuolization. In addition, protein aggregation may occur in the endoplasmic reticulum, with a simultaneous reduction in the expression of BiP chaperones involved in their folding. The increasing level of ROS disrupts the function and structure of mitochondria, including the continuity of the mitochondrial crests and the inner membrane. The dysfunction also affects lysosomes, and its main manifestation is the accumulation of the fluorescent pigment lipofuscin. A probable consequence of the failure of these organelles is also the appearance of β-galactosidase activity in the cytoplasm, which, unlike the so-called complete variant of this enzyme, detected at pH 4.0, is detected at pH 6.0, earning the name "senescence-associated β-galactosidase;

SA-β-Gal). Currently, despite some criticism, SA-β-Gal is the most frequently used marker of old cells in in vitro and in vivo studies. Other recognized markers of old cells are the phosphorylated form of histone H2A.X (γ-H2A.X), specialized domains of facultative heterochromatin (senescence-associated heterochromatic foci; SAHF), DNA-SCARS domains (DNA segments with heterochromatin alterations reinforcing senescence) and a product of oxidative DNA damage, 8-hydroxy-2'-deoxyguanosine (8-OH-dG).

Another important feature of old cells is the change in the expression of many genes that control basic aspects of cell metabolism. At the same time, it should be emphasized that despite morphological degeneration, permanent inability to divide, and extensive, irreparable damage to macromolecules, especially DNA, old cells remain alive and metabolically active for a long time, and their resistance to pro-apoptotic signals plays an important role.

The importance of cell aging for the aging of the body

The first to suggest that cellular aging may reflect specific aspects of the aging of the body as a whole was Leonard Hayflick. The basis for this was the observation that cells collected from mature donors have lower proliferative capabilities than those collected from fetuses. A similar correlation between the age of the donor and the number of cell divisions achieved was observed in cells of the peritoneal mesothelium, vascular endothelium, and keratinocytes. Another proof of the existence of a correlation between cell aging in vitro and the aging of the organism as a whole in vivo was the finding of an increased percentage of old cells in the tissues of elderly people.

The presence of cells with phenotypic features of aging has been demonstrated in the peritoneal cavity, in blood vessels, within atherosclerotic plaques, in the skin, in the cornea, and in intervertebral discs. The accumulation of old cells in tissues, which through their specific secretory profile influence the formation of the local microenvironment, may be the cause of the so-called age-associated degenerative phenotype, which results in increased susceptibility of the body to the development of specific pathologies, including cardiovascular diseases, neurodegenerative diseases and diseases of the musculoskeletal system. This is possible in the face of statistical data that show that the universal, but not obligatory, effects of aging include: progressive muscle atrophy, loss of skin elasticity, prolongation of the average wound healing time, progressive retinal atrophy, and decreased transparency of the lens. eye.

One of the direct effects caused by the presence of old cells in vivo is the disruption of normal tissue structure. This is proven, among others, by research by Parrinello et al., who, analyzing the process of differentiation of breast epithelial cells, showed that the presence of old fibroblasts has a destructive effect (by increasing the secretion of metalloproteases) on the proper formation of branched alveolar structures involved in milk production. However, the accumulation of old pulmonary artery smooth muscle cells in patients with chronic obstructive pulmonary disease turned out to be positively correlated with the development of vascular wall hypertrophy. These cells stimulated the proliferation and migration of their young counterparts, which, according to the authors of the cited work, maybe the basis for the development of pulmonary hypertension in these patients. Old cells may also contribute to the development or exacerbation of atherosclerosis. It is suspected that one of the effects of SASP generated by old cells within the atherosclerotic plaque may be the intensification of the pro-inflammatory environment initially created by macrophages in the subendothelial space.

Aging and the development of cancer

However, the most serious pathology that is inextricably linked to the aging process is cancer. Evidence confirming the existence of a relationship between these two processes comes from both animal experiments and observations of cancer patients. Already in the 1980s Zimmerman et al., analyzing the effect of age on the development of pancreatic tumors in mice, found that exposure of animals to the carcinogenic nitrosourea derivative induces the development of tumors only in older individuals. Studies on a rat model showed that syngeneic transplantation of transformed hepatocytes resulted in the development of cancer lesions primarily in the liver of elderly individuals. In humans, the incidence of cancer increases exponentially with age and affects over 60% of people over 65 years of age. Importantly, a particular acceleration in the rate of cancer development is observed only in adulthood (approximately half of the average human lifespan), which is probably due to the time necessary for the accumulation of a critical number of oncogenic mutations in cells. However, genetic aberrations present in preneoplastic cells, and often also in the adjacent normal cells, do not always translate into the development of a cancer phenotype in vivo. This means that in many types of cancer, the accumulation of a large number of mutations is not a sufficient condition to initiate the proliferation process, which indicates that the appropriate tissue microenvironment is also crucial for tumor progression, allowing the transformation of preneoplastic cells into cells with fully expressed characteristics. malignancy.

Based on information about the accumulation of old cells with age, a concept was developed according to which old cells, especially fibroblasts, can create pro-cancer conditions in the tissue environment. This theory assumes a certain duality of the biological significance of the cellular aging process, which on the one hand, especially in young organisms, may constitute a form of a tumor suppressor mechanism (cells that do not divide cannot undergo cancerous transformation), and on the other, as they accumulate in tissues with age, may promote various elements of cancer progression, especially based on SASP. Direct evidence confirming the pro-cancer effect of old cells was provided by the research of Krtolica et al., who proved that old fibroblasts promote the proliferation of preneoplastic epithelial cells and very aggressive MDA-231 breast cancer cells in vitro to a much greater extent than young cells. The effect also occurred in vivo, when the development of cancer tumors after implanting mixtures of breast cancer cells with old fibroblasts into mice was more intense compared to individuals in which cancer cells were implanted in the presence of young fibroblasts. The authors of the cited work identified direct normal cell-cancer cell interactions as the main mechanism underlying the pro-tumor effect of old fibroblasts. Liu et al. showed that old fibroblasts can stimulate the progression of breast cancer cells in vitro and in vivo also through factors secreted into the environment, including metalloproteases and hepatocyte growth factor (HGF). The combined involvement of cell-cell interactions and factors secreted into the environment (especially amphiregulin) was demonstrated by Bavik et al., who observed the stimulating effect of old fibroblasts on the proliferation of transformed prostate epithelial cells.

Old cells can also indirectly influence the progression of cancer, e.g. by stimulating the phenomenon of angiogenesis, which is fundamental for tumor development. Old fibroblasts turned out to be a strong source of pro-angiogenic factors, which by secreting increased amounts of VEGF effectively increased the degree of invasiveness of vascular endothelial cells through basement membranes. The pro-angiogenic effect of old cells was confirmed by experiments on animals, where increased vascularization of cancer lesions was found after implantation of transformed epithelial cells with old fibroblasts.

6

Eternal youth: how to deceive the genes of old age

The genetics of aging and life expectancy is one of the fundamental disciplines in the study of aging processes. This is where advances in the biology of aging began, since in the early 1990s Cynthia Kenyon from the University of Southern California (USA) showed that a mutation in just one gene in a model animal—the round nematode C. elegans—leads to increasing his life expectancy by 2 times. This fact has allowed many researchers to believe that aging can indeed be significantly slowed down and this can be done here and now.

Since then, research has continued, and other model animals have been added to nematodes: Drosophila fruit flies (a favorite and well-studied object by geneticists) and mice. Thanks to the use of transgenesis methods, all of them have also become actively used in studies of the genetics of aging. If in Cynthia Kenyon's experiment, there was a mutation that turned off the activity of a certain gene product, then transgenesis allows us to study how, on the contrary, the activation of additional copies of certain genes can affect life expectancy and the rate of aging.

Here the most convenient model system turned out to be Drosophila fruit flies since their life expectancy is very short.

Experiments with them made it possible to discover dozens of life expectancy genes.

It turned out that genes associated with aging are mostly associated with the regulation of metabolism and the cell's response to nutrient deficiency. Nutrients are nutrients, such as amino acids, that are needed to build the cellular proteins that keep us alive. Genes associated with the detection of nutrients encode, first of all, various kinases (a type of enzyme - Forbes), which activate the processes of cell growth and division, but at the same time, due to the intensification of metabolism, the number of errors increases, the cell ages faster, and the body as a whole - Same. Therefore, mutations in genes involved in the regulation of metabolism and accelerating it lead to slower aging and increased life expectancy.

A well-known example is the mTOR kinase. It is at the center of metabolic pathways that, in response to the presence of amino acids in the cell, trigger the processes of protein synthesis, and ultimately cell growth and division. But at the same time, this kinase turns off the mechanisms for cleansing the cell from intracellular debris as unnecessary. Autophagy is a phenomenon when a cell begins to digest itself, primarily destroying damaged mitochondria and protein aggregates. This slows down aging. When the cell has enough nutrients, it does not need to turn on the energy-consuming process of self-digestion. Therefore, the aging process accelerates.

Turning off mTOR kinase through mutation or pharmacological inhibition (slowing) leads to the activation of autophagy and the slowdown of aging. An inhibitory effect means suppression of the functions of a specific gene or the protein encoded by that gene. We can turn off the activity of a given gene product pharmacologically when the substance binds to some enzyme, blocks its activity, or sharply reduces it. And if this gene product was involved in the aging process, then we get a slowdown in aging.

Genes that can be classified as longevity genes, on the contrary, are involved in reparative (restorative) processes in the cell, for example, heat shock protein genes. When a cell is stressed, the proteins in it clump into aggregates, which prevents them from performing any function. As a result, the vital activity of the cell slows down (this is bad for the cell and leads to accelerated aging), and heat shock proteins are activated, which pull apart these aggregates or send them for disposal (autophagy).

If transgenesis was previously actively used in simple model animals, such as Drosophila and nematodes, now more expensive and time-consuming studies are increasingly being carried out when transgenesis is carried out in mice. Mice are already mammals; they are evolution-arily close to humans, so such studies are especially valuable. But experiments with mice last for years. However, the results of such studies are preclinical tests, the results of which can be used in medical practice.

If we know the target gene, we can try to regulate its activity during normal aging, including in the human body.

This can be either pharmacological regulation, when substances are selected that inhibit the function of the product, say, an aging-associated gene or, conversely, turn off the inhibitor of the longevity gene. This is a pharmacological path that ultimately leads to the creation of geroprotectors - pharmacological drugs that slow down aging.

However, gene therapy is already on the way, when we will be able to control the function of a gene in the human body, introducing, for example, an additional copy and activating it in some target tissue. Using a gene therapy approach, we will be able to slow down the aging process of blood vessels to overcome atherosclerosis, slow down heart failure, and fight Alzheimer's or Parkinson's disease. It is cardiovascular, metabolic, and neurodegenerative age-related diseases that are the main causes of mortality today.

Over the past couple of decades, the genetics of aging and lifespan have made it possible to identify more than a thousand target genes associated with aging and longevity. A number of these target genes encode proteins for which pharmacological regulators are known. For example, the already mentioned mTOR kinase has a substance called rapamycin as an inhibitor. It has been shown that the addition of rapamycin can lead to an increase in life expectancy in mice by up to 25%.

Unfortunately, not all targets are pharmacologically accessible, and not all are regulated by certain substances, but gene therapy can help here. There are already two studies on mice where, with the help of gene therapy, their life expectancy increased by 22%. Another experiment showed that the introduction of the telomerase gene (an additional copy of the gene for the enzyme that completes the ends of chromosomes) also very significantly extended the life of mice. That is, those targets that are pharmacologically inaccessible, we will in the future be able to regulate using gene therapy.

55

7

Essence of Longevity

Centenarians are considered to be people aged 90 years and above. At the same time, the average age of longevity is 115 years, and scientists still place the absolute theoretical limit at 125 years.

However, recently, researchers have insisted that those who have celebrated their 100th anniversary should be considered centenarians - people's life expectancy is steadily increasing, and the chances of living to the cherished mark are significantly increasing.

How to live 100 years

Human health and longevity depend on many reasons. The most important factors for longevity are:

- genetics
- lifestyle (including nutrition, physical activity and psychological regime, bad and good habits)
- ecology and state of the environment

- healthcare in the country of residence

Scientists have not yet come to a consensus on how much the influence of each factor is expressed in percentage terms. For example, according to various estimates, genetic status is assigned from 8 to 30%, and the importance of image and lifestyle can reach 60%.

It is important to understand that these factors do not contradict each other, but complement and strengthen. Knowing, for example, about genetically reduced protection from the effects of exhaust gases, you will not choose to live in an industrial metropolis and thereby increase your chances of healthy longevity. Or you won't use plastic utensils if you know that your body is susceptible to the toxic effects of bisphenol A, which is part of houschold plastic.

What influences natural longevity

Of the four main factors for longevity that we listed earlier, only genetic characteristics are considered uncontrollable factors. The remaining three can and should be changed.

For example, the World Health Organization has compiled a list of the causes of the most serious diseases that significantly affect the shortening of life. There are 9 of them in total:

1. Hypertension
2. Obesity,
3. High cholesterol levels,
4. Lack of physical activity,
5. Bad habits (smoking, alcohol),
6. Drug use,

7. Unprotected sex,
8. Poor water quality,
9. Contaminated air.

Here we return to the topic of genetics again. Human DNA contains many genes that influence health and potential for longevity. A comprehensive DNA test (e.g.MyExpert) will reveal exactly how vulnerable you are to these nine reasons.

A tendency to high blood pressure or weight gain, impaired alcohol metabolism, or the risk of atherosclerosis are all hereditary factors that are important to identify as early as possible. After all, the genetic profile does not change with age, and if a baby is found to be at risk of developing a particular disease, he will not "grow out." However knowing this will allow you to adjust your lifestyle and diet and prevent the development of the disease.

Genes for longevity

So, do longevity genes exist, or should the reasons for longevity be found in lifestyle and diet? Scientists' research and debate on this topic have not stopped for many years.

On the one hand, studies are showing that following the principles of a healthy diet reduces mortality by 15%. This conclusion was reached by scientists from the Japanese National Center for Global Health and Medicine, who studied the nutrition and lifestyle of 36.6 thousand men and 42.9 thousand women aged 45 to 75 years who had never had cancer for 15 years. stroke, chronic diseases of the cardiovascular system or liver.

On the other hand, no one is in a hurry to deny the influence of heredity. In 2021, scientists from the Joint Institute for Nuclear Research Elena Kravchenko and Anastasia Ivanova received a patent for a "Method for determining the presence of a genetic predisposition to human longevity." According to their assumptions, variants AA and AG of the FOXO3A gene indicate a person's genetic predisposition to longevity and increase his chances of living to 100 years by 1.5 times. However, the GG genotype will not provide such an opportunity. However, these data have not yet been confirmed.

What do human health and longevity depend on?

We have already mentioned the main factors of longevity. This is, first of all, nutrition and lifestyle. If your goal is to be on the list of long-livers, try:

1. Eat a balanced diet. Choose a diet similar to the Mediterranean (rich in fish and seafood, herbs, and vegetables), and adhere to the "plate rule": approximately 50% vegetables and an average of 25% protein and slow carbohydrates.
2. Be physically active. Don't strive for Olympic records, but regularly give your body aerobic exercise.

Let's consider some more factors of human longevity:

1. Proper sleep and rest;
2. Sunbathing with all precautions
3. Psychological comfort and health. Try to avoid chronic stress and negative emotions.
4. Interpersonal relationships and social integration. Man is a collective being, so regular meetings with family, and friends and

a pleasant social environment should become the rule. It is also useful to engage in charity work and volunteer work;

5. Brain activity. The brain's ability to solve complex problems often deteriorates with age, reducing the quality of life affecting overall energy tone, and leading to the development of diseases. Pay attention to neurotics - a physical and cognitive exercise that develops the brain and maintains its activity.

6. Discipline. It sounds strange that people with a high level of responsibility and self-organization most often maintain good physical shape and stable weight, which means they avoid many health problems.

According to medical researchers, the lifespan of the heart is 150 years, the kidneys - 150-200 years, the brain can work for about the same amount of time, and the liver can easily last 600 years. So let's use these resources correctly!

8

Rules of Health and Longevity

Love your life

I t is very important to live an interesting life, to love yourself and those around you, and to find new interests at every stage of your life's journey. With age, a person changes and the life around him changes. First of all, this concerns the physical condition of a person, his financial situation, career (retirement), and position in society.

Therefore, a person needs to find internal resources in himself in order to adapt to a new period in his life - impending old age. The whole point is just who you will become - a youthful old man or a young man aged early. But if you love life and you care about what will happen next, what will happen to your children, grandchildren, friends and loved ones, you have a chance to live a long and fulfilling life.

Because the very desire for longevity makes a person stronger and more resilient and, most importantly, more intelligent and rational. And what is equally important, people who are satisfied with their lives suffer less from colds and cancer than those for whom the light of a happy life seems only a deceptive beacon.

Strive to be creative

This will help you keep your interest in life. Life interests change at different periods of a person's life. And if a person at some stage of his life fails to fully realize himself, he loses interest in life. And only creativity and what he loves helps him maintain interest and love for life. Although creativity can be different (from high art to work in a personal plot), the main thing is that it brings you joy and happiness and makes you young. If you are purposeful and you have a favorite thing that is the meaning of your life, then you are a happy person. Because you have found a worthy occupation for yourself and found your place in life. Creativity will always be an inexhaustible source of interest and love in life. It will distract you from the negative manifestations in life and will help you overcome all sorts of obstacles on your life path. Therefore, under no circumstances should you live in the past, because this often leads to depression. It is necessary that a person, in the conditions of impending old age, devote himself to a favorite activity, an unfinished book or improvement of a dacha, helping relatives, etc. The main thing is that he finds his meaning of life in this . This helps a person live a long and fulfilling life.

Maintain good physical shape.

Laziness and passivity always carry a hidden danger to health, as they are the most common cause of physical inactivity. As a person ages, motor activity usually decreases. This is due to a change in his behavior, the emergence of new habits: sleeping in the afternoon, sitting on the sofa all day and watching TV, avoiding any physical activity moving little, etc. Physical inactivity, combined with excess weight and smoking, accelerates the development of atherosclerosis and makes it heavier. the course of age-related diseases and therefore contributes to premature aging of the body.

If at a young age an increase in physical activity can still compensate for the pathogenic effect of excess weight, then with age, due to physical inactivity and a decrease in muscle mass, there is a risk of developing cardiovascular diseases and type II diabetes mellitus. Decreased muscle activity and muscle wasting may contribute to insulin resistance. On the contrary, in actively training athletes, tissue sensitivity to insulin increases, and consequently, blood sugar levels decrease. This helps normalize carbohydrate metabolism and the course of atherosclerosis.

Therefore, if you do not want to be a hostage to physical inactivity, change your lifestyle and become a physically active person. First, change the way you think about yourself. Imagine that you are strong and energetic. Behave as you did when you were young: dance, sing, meet friends, travel, walk until the morning, give up the sofa and TV, walk more. If you don't have the opportunity to go to the gym, then you can replace it with walks in the fresh air, working in your garden, dancing or cycling. Gradually increase physical activity: give up the elevator, try to climb stairs, use public transport as little as possible. And active rest is a panacea for depression and physical inactivity. A beautiful body is always relevant, this applies not only to poor women driven by diets and training, but also to men who are content with their "beer bellies".

Find the strength to give up bad habits and lead a healthy lifestyle

Much is known about the destructive effects of alcohol and smoking on the human body. And for any sane person it is quite obvious that it is impossible to live a long and healthy life while drinking alcohol and smoking. Therefore, it is very important to realize the harmfulness of bad habits and move on to a healthier lifestyle. As with losing weight, you need to take the first step towards a new life, without putting it off until tomorrow, and give up bad habits now. It's never too late to start a new life. Even if it seems to you that you have completely destroyed your body by overeating, drinking and smoking, you still have a chance to change everything for the better.

Learn to control your diet and maintain a normal weight

In order to properly control your diet, a person needs to follow the main rule of normal eating behavior: eat at a certain time and in a certain place (at home, at work, in the dining room). Avoid casual meals in cafes, eateries, or in the company of friends. It is also necessary to get rid of the pathological stereotype, the habit of relieving emotional stress with food, which is especially typical for beautiful female representatives. Learn to distinguish between hunger and a bad mood and give up the habit of lifting your mood with food and eating only when you are hungry.

It is necessary to control your weight and maintain it within normal limits through exercise and limiting high-carbohydrate foods. To determine your excess weight, you need to calculate the difference between your actual weight and your ideal weight based on your height and build. The best known is Brock's formula, according to which the ideal body weight in kilograms is equal to height in centimeters minus 100. For example, with a height of 160 cm, your normal weight should be 60 kg (160-100 = 60). If your actual weight is 90 kg, then the excess weight is 30 kg (90-60 = 30).

There is a fairly common expression among doctors: "All diseases are caused by excess weight." In fact, take a look at your diet and eating habits, and you may wonder how much you are willing to help your body maintain longevity and youth. And we wish you patience and willpower on the path to good health and beautiful youth.

9

Psychological aspects of Aging

Aging is not only an inevitable biological stage, but also an entry into a new social stage, where it is important not to lose your positive qualities and accept upcoming changes with wisdom. Aging is caused not only by physical changes, but also by deeply psychological ones. They, in turn, can have a serious impact on a person's lifestyle and appearance.

Aging as a psychosomatic process

Psychosomatics is a science that studies the influence of emotions on the body and the development of various diseases. Nature has established that the human body, starting from the age of 25, physically begins to slowly but surely fade away. This is a natural biological process, but individual characteristics of a person can bring this new period closer.

The manifestation of chronic negative emotions, for example, anxiety, stress, suppressed unspoken aggression, have a serious impact on a person's internal and external health:

1. wrinkles and age spots appear
2. Pressure rises
3. Damage to the heart and blood vessels
4. The rate of gray hair appearance increases
5. The body's defense mechanisms are suppressed
6. Elomeres are shortened (sections of chromosomes whose length is directly related to life expectancy)
7. The number of free radicals increases (and, as a result, oxidative stress increases).
8. The level of the longevity hormone – Klotho – decreases (its reduction directly affects the occurrence of atherosclerosis and osteoporosis).
9. Conventionally, we can distinguish 3 types of old age: physical (decreased activity and various diseases), social (limited contacts) and psychosomatic.

If we talk in more detail about the last aspect, then its striking features include:

1. Lack of positive emotions. To feel comfortable, it is periodically important for a person to receive approval of his strengths from others. In science, this term is called "psychological stroking." And a person needs nourishment with new emotions and impressions no less than vitamins.
2. Negative destructive thoughts
3. Self-flagellation
4. Feelings of guilt, inferiority, unfulfillment
5. Self-hypnosis associated with future negative events
6. Manipulation of others using a non-existent disease
7. "Childish" behavior

Physical, social and psychosomatic old age may not coincide with each other. Their greater or lesser manifestation depends on a person's lifestyle, level of intelligence, desire to develop and not give up.

Emotions

Emotions are one of the basic mental functions that allow a person to adapt to new environmental conditions. They can both give confidence and cause apathy. Since the period of aging is in most cases perceived as a negative stage, the emotional sphere also begins to deform: new knowledge and skills are more difficult to understand, adaptive capacity decreases, more free time appears, and a conflict occurs between a person's desires and his capabilities.

Emotional development, even at the initial stage of aging, plays no less important function than intellectual development. We can talk about the emotional degradation of an adult when he is unable to:

1. Recognize and express your emotions;
2. Regulate emotional state;
3. Be aware of the influence of your emotions on other people and vice versa;
4. Take responsibility for your emotions (and instead shift the blame to others);
5. Pay more attention to positive rather than negative emotions.

Scientific research shows that until the later stages of ontogenesis, the parts of the brain responsible for emotions do not undergo critical changes. But, of course, age adjusts their dynamics. For example, aging people try to avoid situations associated with negative emotions; they control their dissatisfaction and anger less diligently than young people but at the same time they tend to assess the situation more sensitively to them.

The influence of mental factors on appearance

Mental factors during the aging process have a direct impact on appearance. Let's consider two personality types - "fighter for life" and "guardian".

"Fighters for life" are active and cheerful people, they are motivated to achieve success and, in spite of everything, find the strength to move forward. Due to the presence of positive emotions, the process of endorphin production occurs. As a rule, in such people the functioning of the immune, antioxidant, and nervous systems is normalized, oxidative stress does not go off scale, and regeneration processes are stably active. Therefore, people of the "fighters for life" type most often look younger than their peers: the stages of gravitational ptosis pass slowly, the skin has a healthy color, it is moisturized and elastic, the network of wrinkles is noticeable, but not deep. Therefore, when such a patient comes to a cosmetologist, correcting aesthetic defects is not a problem.

"Keepers of the past" are people who are fixated on the past, do not want to develop and learn something new, they reflect on old memories and do not want to see prospects in the future. Without knowing it, they begin to activate the mechanism of biological aging. Often such people are irritable, quick-tempered, do not control the flow of negative thoughts and words, limit social contacts and prefer to be alone with themselves. Because of this, the facial muscles are always tense, the eyebrows are furrowed, the complexion takes on a grayish tint and a tired appearance, facial wrinkles are pronounced, and fat packets are thinned. Internal imbalance provokes unwanted external changes, and the result is a vicious circle that can be broken by the joint work of a psychologist and a cosmetologist.

Markers of psychological old age

Psychological age includes the totality of a person's subjective feelings of his age, behavior and actions. Therefore, very often the psychological age does not coincide at all with the mark in the passport. Some even at 70 years old find hobbies, enjoy life, explore the unknown, while others, after 30 years, begin to age with incredible force.

Psychologists have identified markers of psychological old age, thanks to which a person can understand that his energy is directed not in a creative, but in a destructive direction.

Here they are:

Relationships with time.

The first indicator is the thought that all interesting events are behind us and that there is nothing attractive in the future. Psychologically, a young man is not afraid to make plans, while an old man lives only in memories, slowing down his development.

Attitude towards your limitations.

Psychological old age occurs when a person puts self-pity and limitations at the forefront ("I will never...", "I no longer have the strength," "I should have done it earlier"). Psychologically, a young man believes in his strengths and capabilities at any age.

Degree of development of emotional competence.

Emotional competence is the ability to "switch" from oneself to other people, not to judge, and to experience feelings of gratitude. It has been proven that kind and cheerful people have different hormonal and neurochemical processes, thanks to which the face does not become "senile" for a long time.

Thus, the main psychological problem of aging is associated with a personal crisis and determining one's place in life. Those who perceive aging not as the end, but as a new stage in life, lead an active life, and their emotional background is not subject to serious cataclysms. But if you or your relative are prone to reflecting on the past, then it is important to connect additional levels of care from loved ones, and sometimes professional psychological help.

10

Cognitive Impairment

As we age, the brain structures that regulate mood and intellectual processes are the first to change. People around him notice that the person has "gone in": he has become forgetful, touchy, irritable, and sometimes aggressive. Until recently, this was considered normal, because "old age cannot be cured." However, medicine has changed its mind about cognitive impairment in older people. Now there are many drugs with different mechanisms of action that help slow down brain aging. Neuroprotectors of peptide origin take pride of place in this group of drugs.

Isolated cognitive impairment occurs with limited damage to certain parts of the cerebral cortex as a result of stroke, traumatic brain injury, brain tumor, or other causes. And in old age, most chronic progressive brain diseases are accompanied by multiple cognitive disorders, when there is simultaneous suppression of several, and in severe cases, all cognitive functions.

Cognitive Impairment: Mild to Severe

The assessment of cognitive impairment remains challenging. On the one hand, doctors and relatives believe that memory loss, absent-mindedness, and bad mood are the "age-related norm." On the other hand, a doctor does not always have the opportunity to use special, accurate methods for identifying cognitive impairment and determining its severity. Moreover, classifications are constantly revised as knowledge accumulates about the causes of brain disorders.

With the syndrome of severe cognitive impairment, a person completely or partially loses independence and independence. This may be the case, in particular, with dementia of a degenerative or vascular nature. It forms when there is significant damage to the brain, which usually develops over a long period. According to epidemiological data, at least 5% of people over 65-70 years old suffer from dementia.

Moderate cognitive impairment goes beyond the average age norm. They do not cause maladjustment, although they can lead to difficulties in difficult and unusual situations for the patient. In older adults, the prevalence of mild cognitive impairment is 11–17%. Over a 5-year follow-up period, moderate cognitive impairment transformed into severe in half of the patients.

Mild cognitive impairment is said to occur when a function declines from its baseline level. They do not affect daily life and work. In any case, you need to pay attention to them, because mild cognitive impairment may signal an early stage of organic brain damage.

Before Sunset: Non-Dementia Disorder

Dementia (dementia) is most often the result of a long-term process in the brain. Although it can also be a consequence of traumatic brain injury, encephalitis, stroke, or intoxication. In most cases, cognitive impairment and dementia are interrelated—cognitive impairment appears first but does not reach the level of dementia, and then dementia develops. That is why in recent years more and more attention has been paid to non-dementia (early) forms of cognitive impairment. Timely diagnosis of these disorders and their treatment can delay or even prevent the onset of dementia.

Alzheimer's Disease

This is the most common form of dementia and is neurodegenerative. People over 65 years of age are more likely to get sick. To date, the cause of the disease has not been clarified. Modern methods of therapy only slightly mitigate the symptoms, but do not yet allow either stopping or slowing down the development of the disease.

Vascular Dementia and Encephalopathies

Vascular lesions of the brain are the second most common cause of dementia in the elderly.

Causes of vascular dementia:

1. Brain injury
2. Diabetes
3. Vegetative-vascular dystonia
4. Chronic brain starvation

5. Drug addiction
6. Hypertonic disease
7. Radiation exposure

As a rule, the development of vascular dementia is preceded by dyscirculatory encephalopathy with cognitive impairment. The main damaging factor is brain hypoxia. Discirculatory encephalopathy is characterized by gradual development with periodic temporary improvements.

In the initial stages you may be concerned about:

1. Headache,
2. Feeling of heaviness ("fog") in the head,
3. Dizziness,
4. Episodes of coordination,
5. Insomnia,
6. Emotional ability,
7. Irritability,
8. Increased fatigue.

Also possible are minor memory impairments and "sharpening" of certain character traits (grumpiness, stinginess, fussiness). Dementia due to vascular encephalopathy develops quite often unless death occurs from a stroke or cardiovascular disease. Differential diagnosis is carried out with alcoholic and dysmetabolic encephalopathy.

Treatment Of Cognitive Impairment In Old Age

It has 2 main goals: slowing the progression of the disease and reducing the severity of existing disorders.

Before starting treatment, it is necessary to comprehensively examine the patient. Without this, achieving the maximum possible compensation for cardiovascular and other somatic diseases is impossible. It is necessary to try to reduce vascular risk factors as much as possible: arterial hypertension, hyperlipidemia, and obesity. Regular intake of statins and antiplatelet drugs and physical activity are required. As a rule, patients have depression of varying severity. In this case, antidepressants recommended in geriatric practice are prescribed.

Treatment has two directions:

1. optimization of microcirculation and cerebral metabolic processes
2. optimization of synaptic transmission processes.

Neuroprotectors of peptide nature "work" in both directions. On the one hand, they regulate the ratio of inhibitory and excitatory amino acids in brain structures and also normalize the level of mediators (substances that are involved in the transfer of nervous excitation from one nerve cell to another). On the other hand, they have a positive effect on metabolic processes in the brain. Therefore, such drugs have become an integral part of the complex treatment of cognitive impairment at all stages: from mild encephalopathies to severe dementia.

11

The Science of Longevity. What technologies can extend life

The global anti-aging market is $110 billion, and according to Bank of America forecasts, it will grow to $610 billion by 2025. Hundreds of companies annually invest a lot of money in developments that should slow down aging or eliminate its consequences: from stem cell research and senolytics to prevent Alzheimer's and Parkinson's diseases. In 2021, San Diego-based Human Longevity raised $330 million in investments to develop technology that, based on a person's genetic data, will generate recommendations to increase his life expectancy. New York-based Elysium Health has raised more than $70 million to turn scientific advances into consumer products. Its latest product is a dietary supplement to improve cellular aging. Some countries have even created political parties that support progress in life extension, such as the US Transhumanist Party. But are there any real scientific achievements in this area?

The underlying assumption of a business built on aging is that the process can be slowed down. At first glance, this seems plausible. Compared to previous generations, we are living longer: since the mid-

1800s, the maximum human lifespan has increased by 3 months every year. But in the summer of 2021, the British scientific journal Nature Communications published an article by an international group of scientists, according to which the rate of human aging does not change and cannot yet be slowed down due to biological limitations and the lack of methods to overcome them. The rate of aging refers to the rate at which mortality increases with age. Scientists compared the ages of death of people from different historical eras and different nationalities, as well as 6 genera of primates, both wild and captive. It turned out that the rate of aging in humans and animals is fairly constant, with minor differences between populations.

The rate of human aging has not changed since the 1800s, but people are now living longer due to social, economic, and health improvements. Previously, there were difficult living and working conditions and there was no access to medicine. As a result, many people died young. A further significant increase in human life expectancy will depend on whether technologies appear that can slow down the rate of aging, namely, reduce mortality in old age.

Cure for old age

A "pill for old age" has not yet been invented, because aging itself is not recognized as a disease. Scientists still cannot come to a consensus on this issue, dividing it into two camps: some call to recognize aging as a disease and begin to treat it, and others consider it a natural process since everyone faces it with age. Both have not yet been able to prove their point of view. If aging itself is not considered a disease, then clinical trials of anti-aging drugs cannot be conducted. After all, a medicine is being developed to treat a disease. Before the drug hits the pharmacy shelves, it undergoes a series of serious studies developed according to certain rules and regulations. During this process, the effectiveness and safety of the drug is determined.

Now there are studies of the influence of various methods and substances on the aging of animals, but there are no serious studies of a similar process in humans. It has been shown in many living organisms, from yeast to primates, that caloric restriction in food increases their lifespan. For example, in simple brewer's yeast, which feeds only on carbohydrates in the absence of air access, a decrease in glucose in the environment from 2% to 0.5% increases life expectancy by 25%. At first, this effect was explained by a decrease in the amount of by-products in cells when consuming fewer nutrients: less food means less waste. But then they discovered that the increase in life expectancy occurs due to a decrease in excess mortality from obesity. They tried to test the effect of calorie restriction in people in 2019 and even found a decrease in risk factors for developing cardiovascular diseases with such a diet. However, this study lasted only 2 years, during which it is impossible to conclude the effect on life expectancy. Additionally, the 143 people in the study group were advised to reduce their caloric intake by 25%, but this proved too difficult for most of them and the average calorie reduction in this group over 2 years was only 12%.

Studies of the drugs metformin and rapamycin, already known in fairly wide circles of biohackers, which simulate calorie restriction at the cellular level, are also not sufficient for unambiguous conclusions. Metformin is used to treat type 2 diabetes, and rapamycin is an immunosuppressant used to prevent organ rejection after transplantation. Their effectiveness against these diseases has been tested and proven in clinical studies, but there are no serious studies regarding aging. Therefore, self-administration of these drugs without indications can lead to negative consequences. The same applies to the so-called senolytics. These are drugs that can trigger the death of old cells. Destruction of old cells allows you to get rid of not only non-functioning cells but also those that work to form tumors due to accumulated "errors" in DNA. Most of the senolytics have been tested as anticancer drugs, but not as anti-aging drugs.

Age-related diseases

Although aging itself is not recognized as a disease, drugs can be developed to treat so-called age-related diseases. These are diseases whose frequency increases in old age and which often cause death in older people. These include many types of cancer, neurodegenerative diseases such as Alzheimer's and Parkinson's disease, cardiovascular diseases, atherosclerosis, and type 2 diabetes.

In the science of aging, there is a so-called strategy for achieving negligible aging using engineering methods (SENS). This term was coined by controversial gerontologist Aubrey de Gray to refer to technologies aimed at eliminating the root causes of age-related diseases in 7 areas: neutralization of cancer mutations, elimination of mutations in mitochondrial DNA, cleansing cells of accumulated unnecessary substances, removing intercellular waste, replacing damaged cells, removal of malfunctioning cells, replacement of intercellular polymer bonds. By solving these problems, negligible aging will be achieved where the risk of dying will be constant throughout life, rather than increasing with age. De Gray believes that even without knowing the fundamental causes of aging, it can be dramatically slowed down and made negligible. However, most scientists do not believe in the success of this strategy given the current level of understanding of the causes of aging and the development of medical technologies. We simply do not currently have the knowledge and techniques to do this.

In the fight against age-related diseases, attempts have already been made to use transplantation using animal donor organs. Thus, in January 2022, doctors from the United States announced the first pig heart transplant to a human. 57-year-old American David Bennett Sr. suffered from incurable heart failure and agreed to experimental surgery after he was repeatedly refused to be placed on the waiting list to receive a heart from a human donor. He received a heart transplant from a genetically modified pig created by the biotech company Revivicor. Changes were made to the genome of this animal that contributed to less rejection in humans. But two months after the pioneering transplant, the man died. The cause of death is still unknown, and it is unclear whether Bennett Sr.'s body rejected the pig's heart. Bennett's xenotransplantation (cross-species transplantation) was initially considered successful. For a month after the operation, his body did not reject the animal organ. This period is considered critical for transplant patients. After careful analysis, the results of the post-mortem examination will be published in a peer-reviewed medical journal.

What about gene therapy, which has been actively developing recently? The aging process is complex and not well understood, so there is little hope for creating a gene therapy drug for aging shortly. This field is now evolving towards the development of drugs for the treatment of diseases for which the cause is identified in the form of a specific genetic disorder (and preferably one). For example, in 2019, the gene therapy drug Zolgensma for the treatment of spinal muscular atrophy of the first type in children was approved in the United States, and two years later in Russia, becoming the most expensive drug in the world (the price of one dose is $ 2 million). There is a known cause for this disease: mutations in the SMN1 gene. Therefore, it became possible to develop this drug, which replaces a non-functioning gene.

Internal aging and its external manifestations are strongly connected. It is traditionally believed that wrinkles and excess weight are indispensable companions of old age. Scientists are actively searching for genetic variants that determine skin changes during aging. One of the areas of search was genetic studies of Asian residents, who often look younger than Europeans of the same age. But while certain genetic variants have been identified that differ between Europeans and Asians, the reason for the latter's younger appearance has not yet been determined. Most scientists believe that it has to do with the structure and shape of the face. Having more subcutaneous fat around the eyes and mouth prevents wrinkles from appearing in these areas.

Weight gain after 40 years of age has long been attributed to the slowing of metabolism at this age. However, a study published last year in the scientific journal Science found that this is not the case. Well, at least until the age of 60. Researchers studied data from 6,400 people aged 8 days to 95 years from 29 countries. They were given water to drink in which some of the hydrogen and oxygen were replaced with their labeled varieties (atoms with a radioactive label), which can be detected, for example, in urine, and calculated how much hydrogen and oxygen a person loses per day. And then, using these data, calculate how much carbon dioxide the body produces. This is a very accurate measure of calories burned because a person cannot burn calories without releasing carbon dioxide. Scientists have found that metabolism peaks at age 1, when children burn calories 50% faster than adults, and then gradually decline by about 3% per year until age 20. After this, metabolism does not change until about 60 years of age, when it again begins to slowly decline by 1% annually.

The mechanism of aging is still unknown, and it is not recognized as a disease; realistic prospects for increasing human life expectancy concern methods of reducing mortality from age-related diseases. It is in this direction that most scientists are working and it is in this area that progress is possible.

83

III

The Secrets to Living Your Healthiest Life

12

Lifestyle Choices for Longevity

Accrding to the World Health Organization, there is a trend towards an increase in the proportion of the older generation. This problem is relevant for almost all countries of the world.

The process of population aging depends on many factors: social conditions, labor and physical activity, environmental climate, living conditions, quality of nutrition, and characteristics of the body. Depending on all this, old age can be early, or it can be late.

Aging can be natural, slow, and pathological. Natural aging is the normal course of a person's life and the functioning of his body. Pathological aging is premature aging, when body functions wear out faster and a person ages earlier than his peers. Slow aging is characterized by a slower rate of age-related changes relative to natural aging than in the entire population. This type of aging is the phenomenon of longevity[4].

Life expectancy (longevity) is directly influenced by human health. Longevity is a socio-biological phenomenon, which consists of the fact that a person reaches high age levels.

Health is one of the highest human values, a source of happiness, and joy, and the key to optimal personal fulfillment.

According to the WHO definition, health is a state of a person characterized not only by the absence of disease or physical defects but by complete physical, mental (psychological), and social well-being.

This approach to defining health allows a person to correctly consider his health and use all its capabilities to improve its quality. Therefore, maintaining the health of older people is of great importance for the entire state as a whole.

Health is important for older people because the aging process involves changes not only physically, but also psychologically. Therefore, communication with the elderly has its specifics. In an elderly person, memory is most often impaired, physical activity decreases, anxiety, aggressiveness towards others, and self-doubt appear.

Research by scientists has shown that if every person adhered to the 10 basic rules of a healthy lifestyle, we would live at least 100 years. These 10 tips, developed by an international group of psychologists, doctors, and nutritionists, are as follows:

1. Do only work that pleases you;
2. Always have your point of view;
3. Adhere to the rules of rational nutrition;
4. Give up bad habits;
5. Sleep at a temperature of 17-18°C;

6. Treat everything with love and tenderness;
7. Engage in active mental work;
8. Eat sweets periodically;
9. Give your body emotional relief more often;
10. Do physical labor.

It seems simple, but we love extremes. Some spend half their life sitting on the sofa with the remote control, some eat to their heart's content, and some work until exhaustion, even in their dreams managing to calculate the profitability of the deal. And then even advanced modern medicine cannot save him from illnesses. 50% of a person's health is determined by how healthy a lifestyle he leads, 20% by genetic factors and heredity, another 20% by living conditions (ecology, climate, place of residence), and 10% by healthcare.

Not even one normal person wants to be sick; everyone strives to live a long, happy life. Remember how you strive: barely getting out of bed in the morning, getting ready for school or work in 10 minutes, eating a couple of sandwiches for breakfast, being nervous all day, quarreling with loved ones, envying colleagues and acquaintances, not having time to have a normal lunch, spending the evening at on the couch in front of the TV, watching an advertisement, going to the refrigerator, because at dinner you need to make up for what was missed for breakfast and lunch. Do you think living like this can keep you healthy?

What is meant by the term healthy lifestyle in other countries?

Sweden

For Swedes, taking care of your health is primarily about physical activity. They prefer to walk, take walks, be active, and move until they are old, so old people who can barely walk (but move) do not surprise anyone there. The week of "sports holiday" is also a very healthy tradition. Well, the residents of this country never forget about their two-wheeled friend.

USA

The world leadership in obesity is more revealing than any sociological survey. True, Americans talk to each other about a healthy lifestyle no less often than the British talk about the weather. Their desire to be healthy is also demonstrated by the promotion of smoking, which I began in kindergarten.

China

One of the reports from the Chinese Ministry of Health contained disappointing figures: only 25% of the urban and 10% of the rural population of this country can pay for medical services. But ancient traditions do not allow the Chinese to die out: they move a lot, eat a few harmful foods, know how to quickly, and practice massage and acupuncture almost every day.

Japan

Japanese sociologists, having collected information about the lifestyle and habits of the centenarians of this country, developed their principles of a healthy lifestyle: sleep more, eat less, know how to relax, constantly force your brain to work, know how to laugh, do not dress too warmly, do not drink or smoke. All Japanese want to be healthy, but, unfortunately, they prefer miracle drugs that are constantly advertised on TV over physical activity.

What is a healthy lifestyle?

The concept of "healthy lifestyle" is sociological. The Encyclopedia of Sociology explains it this way:

A healthy lifestyle is a concept of social policy, which is based on the recognition of the high importance of health in society, the responsibility for maintaining health on the part of the individual, state, society, and social group, and asserting the need to take specific actions and measures aimed at creating a favorable and safe environment.

To put it simply, a healthy lifestyle is what allows us, living in an unfavorable environment and stressful situations in a big city, to feel good; this is what allows us to maintain good health and activity into old age.

Healthy lifestyle and proper nutrition.
The food we eat ensures the development of tissues and cells of the body, and their constant renewal, and is also a source of energy. The metabolism in our body depends entirely on the nature of our diet. Our ability to work, morbidity, physical development and growth, neuropsychological state, and life expectancy depend on what we eat. Therefore, proper nutrition and a healthy lifestyle are inseparable.

All nutrition theories try to solve one problem: the intake of sufficient amounts of carbohydrates, fats, proteins, vitamins, microelements, and minerals into the body in the correct proportions. Proper nutrition is based on adherence to the regime (optimally four meals a day with an interval of 4-5 hours between meals); maintaining the caloric intake of the diet (an adult on average needs 3 thousand kcal); the ratio of proteins, fats, carbohydrates (mental work - 1:0.8:3, physical activity - 1:1:5, on average - 1:1:4); covering the body's needs for basic substances (water, trace elements, minerals, vitamins, polyunsaturated fatty acids, amino acids).

Healthy lifestyle and sports.

Movement is life, and active movement is a healthy life. Daily exercise is the key to beauty and health. It is important that sport, in addition to benefits, brings pleasure, and for this, you need to choose the sport that suits you. For a woman, the best sport is regular swimming; for those who lead a sedentary lifestyle, walking or hiking are ideal; jogging at a steady rhythm can be done by the whole family, as well as cycling; in winter, don't forget about skiing and skating. It is important to remember that any sport if approached incorrectly, is traumatic.

To determine how healthy your lifestyle is, take a short test:

1) Do you often eat fresh vegetables and fruits? (yes - 1 point, no - 0 points).

2) Do you try to regularly eat fibrous foods, bran, or thickly ground bread? (yes - 1 point, no - 0 points).

3) Do you love your job? (yes - 1 point, no - 0 points).

4) Do you limit your consumption of animal fats? (yes - 1 point, no - 0

points).

5) Do you limit your sugar intake? (yes - 1 point, no - 0 points).

6) Do you do anything outside of work (hobbies)? (yes - 1 point, no - 0 points).

7) Do you have a person you love? (yes - 1 point, no - 0 points).

8) Are you often bored? (yes – 0 points, no – 1 point).

9) Do you engage in sports that are hazardous to your health? (yes – 0 points, no – 1 point).

10) Do you smoke? (yes – 0 points, no – 1 point).

11) Do you drink alcohol? (yes – 0 points, no – 1 point).

12) Is your weight normal? (yes - 1 point, no - 0 points).

13) Do you often worry or worry about trifles? (yes – 0 points, no – 1 point).

14) Do you do exercises every morning? (yes - 1 point, no - 0 points).

15) Do you take sleeping pills before bed? (yes – 0 points, no – 1 point).

16) Do you often have to buy medicine? (yes – 0 points, no – 1 point).

17) Do you often check your blood pressure? (yes - 1 point, no - 0 points).

18) Can you relax quickly? (yes - 1 point, no - 0 points).

Result:

If you score 17-18 points, you are leading a truly healthy lifestyle, and not just for show. If you scored less, you have something to work on.

The main thing is to always remember: "Your health is in your hands!"

13

Tips for Healthy Lifestyle

A healthy lifestyle is not only correct but also fashionable today. In this chapter, we would like to give 10 basic tips for those who want to start a new healthy, and happy life. They are all simple and yet very important. With the help of these recommendations, you can correct your figure, improve your well-being, feel light, and free your thoughts.

Drink more water

Yes, we forget about clean water. You need to drink at least a liter a day! And tea, coffee, and sweet sodas are not water, moreover. Some of these only harm the body. It is also necessary to periodically visit mineral water pump rooms to drink water rich in beneficial minerals. Don't forget to consult your doctor before doing this.

Proper nutrition

It is necessary not only to get in shape but also to normalize the general condition of the body. We are what we eat. And this is not just a saying. Once you eliminate unhealthy fast food, fatty foods, baked goods, and salty foods from your diet, you will experience significant changes in your well-being. In addition to the lightness that will come literally after a few days of proper nutrition, your sleep and emotional state will improve.

Dream

How much time do you spend sleeping? 4-5 hours? This is not enough for the body to recover. Of course, you can't get rid of fatigue and irritability until you adjust your sleep time. We also recommend replacing the TV with a book. And, of course, don't skimp on a good mattress and pillow.

Active lifestyle

You don't have to run to the gym to lift weights. It's enough to run a couple of kilometers in the evening before going to bed or do your favorite dance. This will not only tighten your muscles but also give you a great mood. Studying at home is also welcome; moreover, just go to the Internet and find suitable video instructions there. But we consider one of the most enjoyable and useful ways to do yoga or gymnastics outdoors, for example, on the Anapa beach. All resorts here have their own clean, guarded beach.

Rest in a sanatorium

It's the most pleasant way to spend a vacation by the sea, so we recommend combining business with pleasure. The best sanatoriums in Anapa offer a variety of treatments based on natural ingredients, for example, mud baths or swimming in indoor pools in Anapa filled with mineral hydrogen sulfide water. Each procedure, of course, is prescribed by a doctor, but many of them are intended not only for treatment but also for the prevention of diseases. Among other things, simply being in a favorable climate will bring incredible benefits.

Rejection of bad habits

A very important point that speaks for itself. And most importantly, remember that your bad habits harm not only you but also your loved ones, primarily children. Think about what step forward you will take for them and yourself by giving up smoking, alcohol, and other things. This is not always easy to do, so psychologists help in this case.

Walks in the open air

What does life consist of on weekdays? Home, transport, work, transport, home. And if the work is sedentary, then it's no good at all. But nothing prevents you from taking a walk in the evening. Yes, even around the house with a dog. Or in the park with friends, loved ones, or children. All this is to our benefit.

Love yourself

Being complex has never helped anyone in life. Accept yourself for who you are, and then start working on improving your already good self. Believe me, people will reach out, love will meet, and success will begin at work. If you still cannot cope with the problem yourself, be sure to consult a psychologist. He will help you find the path to a happy life without complexes and sadness.

Communication with people

We are, of course, talking about positive communication, which can bring pleasure. So, an evening spent with friends can energize you for the whole week. And don't forget about non-verbal communication: touching, hugging, handshaking. All this is very useful for our emotional and physical state, so prefer communication on social media networks - live communication.

Breath

It would seem that what's wrong with this... And this is important Having mastered the technique of diaphragmatic breathing, you can do a lot: control your psycho-emotional state, be able to calm down in a stressful situation, slow down aging, get rid of acne, and much more Unfortunately, we sometimes "forget" to breathe altogether! Yes, yes for example, when we are very concentrated. And at this time the brain requires oxygen.

14

Holistic Approach to Health

A holistic approach to life is becoming more and more popular. More and more people are realizing that the power of nature is far more powerful than all the possible drugs and practices offered to us by conventional healthcare. Perhaps this path is the right option to start anew and carry out a much-needed detox of body and mind. Cleanse yourself of harmful toxins, heal your body physically and mentally, and appreciate what you have. In this chapter, we will answer all your questions and introduce you to the practices that we identify with from a holistic perspective.

What is holism and a holistic approach to life?

Holism is a lifestyle that understands a person as a whole. A holistic approach to life therefore includes taking care of the body, mind, and surrounding environment. It refuses to examine individual functions and parts of the human body separately, as they are closely related and mutually influencing. You can therefore expect comprehensive advice and tips on how to heal and streamline your daily routines and enrich them with functional holistic elements to help you achieve a healthy and long-lasting detox.

Did you know that detox doesn't have to be just about diet?

With the term detox, everyone is guaranteed to imagine fasting or a diet consisting of more or less tasty juices. But it doesn't even start there, and above all, it doesn't even end there. Diet is of course extremely important and, as Hippocrates himself said, all diseases begin in the intestines, but detox can be conducted on several levels :

1. Digital Detox
2. Household detox
3. Detoxification of the organism

We can detoxify ourselves from everything toxic to us:

1. Unhealthy food
2. Chemical preparations
3. Social networks
4. Harmful daily habits
5. Disturbed circadian rhythm
6. Gloomy thoughts
7. The community we surround ourselves with

And since it's a new year, it wouldn't be out of place to give your body a little attention. Come and focus with us on new and perhaps undiscovered paths to a better and more satisfied self. Give nature and pure holistic thoughts a chance.

Digital Detox

Cleaning up from social media and blue light can be harder than it seems. Many of us have a phone almost attached to our hands. But there are many reasons why we should focus on digital detox at least to a small extent. Not only does consuming content on social media often lead to procrastination, but these bad habits also rob us of dopamine (the happy hormone). And sometimes very noticeably. On social networks, we do not only come across educational and beneficial content. We're forced to watch other people's seemingly perfect lives, and that can throw anyone off at times. Even though all online communication channels distribute stress even faster than anything else.

```
The release of dopamine is the very reason people become
addicted.
Social media is like refined sugar. They suddenly increase
the level of dopamine, but in the long term contribute to
its deficiency. Therefore, the brain easily creates the
impression that it cannot exist without social networks.
```

The second pest here is blue light. This very intensively confuses our circadian rhythm, slows down the production of melatonin, and induces in our heads the feeling that it is always daytime, which disrupts one of the most fundamental factors of comprehensive health - sleep. During sleep, the body regenerates, builds immunity, creates energy, and restores that all-important dopamine. Quality sleep should therefore have the same importance in our lives as a quality and varied diet. Without enough energy, no physiological process will function properly. This includes digestion and the function of all detoxification organs.

Digital detox Benefits

- Mental health support
- Work efficiency and overall productivity
- Improving social relationships
- Better sleep
- The ability to focus on yourself

The founder of Blender.cz, ťPeo Chodelka, for example, really enjoys digital detox. He only uses social networks on a work level, he hasn't appeared on them privately for a long time, and for example, you won't see his phone at a joint team building event.

"At the outset, I must say that I still remember the moment when I first realized how much time I was spending on social networks. I was looking through the various settings on the phone and I got to a statistic called Screen Time. These will show you how many hours you spend each day on the phone and in individual applications.

My average Screen Time was almost five hours. Five hours. Of that, an hour a day was Instagram. Yes, I spent one-fifth of the day on my phone and an hour on Instagram. Every single day. It was a similar moment of realization for me as when I stood on the scale a few years ago and it showed 103 kg. I just knew I had to change something.

I uninstalled Facebook, Instagram, and Twitter. I turned off all notifications except SMS. I canceled my personal Instagram account and only used the work one. I reduced the average Screen Time from five hours to two and a half.

And what does that give me? First of all, two and a half hours of extra time every day. It's unbelievable how much time we can spend on our phones and social networks.

I also feel freer that I don't have to share every experience of my real life in the virtual world. Although I still take a lot of photos :)"

Blue light is especially harmful in the evening when the brain should be preparing for sleep.

How to digital detox?

You don't necessarily have to spend days or weeks without your phone. It is abundantly sufficient when you introduce the regime.

1. Don't use your phone as an alarm clock and go without it for at least an hour after waking up.
2. Don't eat with your phone in your hand. Set it aside and enjoy your meal.
3. If you're spending time with friends or family, leave your phone in your pocket and take in your surroundings.
4. While walking in nature, don't check social media or text with friends, don't answer emails, and just observe the environment.
5. Don't take your phone to the toilet.
6. Do not unlock the screen at least 1 hour before going to bed and protect yourself from blue light and distractions.
7. Start using airplane mode when you're not working.

8. Believe that when you get used to the omnipresence of the digital world, you will be relieved.

Household detoxification

It's not called purity half health for nothing. The environment in which we live also largely shapes us. The household should be clean, and organized and you should not group items that you don't use and don't need. The fewer things distract us, the calmer our mind is and it has room for the really important stimuli.

Why should environmental detoxification not be forgotten?

1. Cleaning frees the mind.
2. Cleanliness prevents the formation of mites.
3. The minimalistic and tidy environment does not distract from work.
4. Regular cleaning induces systematicity and clarity.

The state of the household is therefore primarily related to our psychological level. You probably know that moment when you come home tired from work and suddenly see what you still have to do or clean in an environment where you want to rest. But the most common response to this fact is not productivity. It's procrastination and an emotional slump. The irritability caused by the feeling of lack of time then contributes to the deepening of chronic stress. And now you probably know where we're going with this - stress is the main enemy of immunity .

How to detoxify the environment?

1. Clean up your desk and don't leave anything unrelated to work on it.
2. Scrub the kitchen area thoroughly and keep it clean.
3. Organize the food in the fridge. Sealable containers or various waiting lists will serve you well.
4. Remember that the dining table is not a place to store unnecessary things.
5. Sort out unnecessary things and donate them where someone else will use them.
6. Don't keep unnecessary things that you rationally know you will never need.
7. Give space to indoor plants. It oxygenates the air and makes the space cozy.

Detoxification of the organism

The last pillar of detoxification, which we will cover, is body detox. If you decide to do this cleaning as well, we recommend that you find out as much information as possible about it. We will now try to introduce you to detoxification without pretense. We will show you the positives and negatives associated with these processes and list the basic types of detoxes. You can then decide whether it is right for you or not.

"If you feel that detox is just what you need, never do it alone. Take the advice of the experienced or entrust yourself to the care of a specialist. Detox of the organism also brings many pitfalls, which are not good to mess with."

Major detoxification organs include

1. Liver
2. Kidneys
3. Intestines
4. Skin
5. Lymphatic system

These organs are themselves adapted to carry out purification. And they do it without a break. We can help them with this and make their work easier or give them a moment of rest by fasting. There are also processes that you can set up yourself without professional help. But we don't mean drastic changes in the menu or even the already mentioned fasts. You have to be very careful there.

15

Mental Health Tips

In life's challenging journey, mental well-being is a beacon that guides us to balance and self realization. As we navigate the complexities of our daily existence, understanding the basics of mental health becomes paramount. From simple, uplifting joys to deep mindfulness practices, there are many paths to living a balanced life.

Self-awareness

Self-awareness is a deep understanding of your emotions, desires, strengths, and weaknesses. It is the compass that guides our reactions, behavior, and interactions.

Methods for increasing self-awareness

Introspection

1. Devote moments of solitude to reflection.
2. Dive deeply into understanding personal thoughts, feelings, and motivations, promoting a deeper connection with yourself.

Logging

1. A chronicle of daily experiences, emotions, and thoughts.
2. Revisit these entries to witness personal growth and patterns, offering a tangible road map of your emotional journey.

Feedback

1. Welcome ideas from trusted peers and loved ones.
2. Use this external perspective as a mirror reflecting areas of growth and affirmation.

Emotional intelligence:

1. Develop the ability to recognize, understand, and manage personal emotions.
2. Use this understanding to manage your interpersonal relationships with compassion and grace.

Healthy lifestyle

A harmonious balance between physical and mental well-being, where the body and mind support and elevate each other.

Components of a healthy lifestyle

Nutrition

1. Nourish your body with a varied diet rich in essential nutrients.
2. Consume foods that nourish the brain, such as those rich in

omega-3 fatty acids, which improve mood and improve cognitive function.

Physical activity

1. Fill your daily routine with movement, whether it's a relaxing walk in nature or an invigorating workout.
2. Notice the release of endorphins, the body's natural mood enhancers, increasing both physical and mental vitality.

Sleep

1. Cherish sleep as a sacred ritual to rejuvenate your mind and body.
2. Create a serene environment and sleep rhythm, ensuring your body gets the rest and recovery it needs.

Humidification

1. Quench your body's thirst with plenty of water, supporting every cellular function.
2. Recognize the key role of hydration in maintaining cognitive acuity and overall vitality.

Stress management

In today's dynamic and constantly evolving world, stress has become an almost inevitable part of life. Effectively managing this stress is critical to mental balance and overall well-being.

Meditation

A practice that centers the mind and calms the spirit. Through focused breathing and mindfulness, meditation can reduce anxiety, improve self-awareness, and promote emotional health.

Deep breathing exercises

These are simple yet powerful techniques that can be practiced anywhere. Taking deep, controlled breaths can activate the body's relaxation response, reducing stress and increasing feelings of calm.

Hobbies

Engaging in activities that bring you joy and passion can be a natural antidote to stress. Whether it's painting, reading, gardening, or any other hobby, it provides an opportunity to take a break from everyday worries and rejuvenate.

Time management and organization

A chaotic environment or schedule can increase feelings of stress. By organizing tasks, setting priorities, and managing time effectively, you can create a structured and less stressful daily routine.

Stay in touch

At their core, humans are social creatures. We thrive on interaction, understanding, and sharing. Creating and maintaining meaningful connections is vital to emotional and mental well-being.

Interaction with loved ones

Spending quality time with family and friends can provide comfort, understanding, and a sense of belonging. These moments, whether in everyday conversations or special occasions, strengthen our emotional well-being.

Community participation

Participating in community events, volunteering, or attending local meetings can help build connections and a sense of purpose. Being part of a community offers support and the feeling that you are part of something larger than yourself.

Joining clubs and organizations

Whether it's a book club, sports team, or hobby group, joining organizations that align with personal interests can provide regular social interaction and a platform to meet like-minded people.

Support systems

During difficult times, having a strong support system becomes invaluable. Formed by close friends, family, or support groups, this system offers guidance, understanding, and a listening ear when it is needed most.

Limit your substance use

Substances, whether legal such as alcohol or illegal drugs, can have a significant impact on a person's mental and emotional well-being. Over-reliance or misuse can lead to a variety of medical and social problems.

Alcohol consumption

Although many cultures and societies perceive alcohol as a social lubricant, it is important to understand its effects on the brain and body. Excessive alcohol consumption can impair judgment, increase feelings of depression, and lead to addiction.

Illegal drugs

Using illicit drugs or misusing prescription medications can have serious mental health consequences. They can change brain chemistry, lead to addiction, and worsen mental health problems.

Awareness and moderation

Being aware of your consumption and setting limits is vital. Moderation will ensure that you don't cross the line from occasional use to addiction.

Looking for help

Recognizing when substance use becomes problematic is critical. Professional help, whether counseling, rehabilitation, or support groups, can provide guidance and resources for recovery.

Set boundaries

Boundaries delineate personal space, both physically and emotionally. These are the invisible lines that determine how a person interacts with others and how they allow others to interact with them.

Personal relationships

In personal relationships, boundaries can define emotional availability, personal space, or even topics of conversation. They provide mutual respect and understanding

Professional settings

In the workplace, boundaries may be related to workload, working hours, or interpersonal interactions. Setting clear professional boundaries ensures a healthy work-life balance and prevents burnout.

Communication

Setting clear boundaries is important. It's not just about installing them; it's about being understood and respected by others.

Self-care and relaxation

Boundaries also apply to yourself. Making time for self-care, relaxation, and personal activities promotes mental well-being and prevents feelings of overwhelm.

Seek professional help

In a world where mental health problems are becoming increasingly common, seeking professional advice is not only wise but often necessary. It is a sign of strength and self-awareness to recognize when external experience is required.

Therapists and consultants

These professionals are trained to help people cope with emotional and psychological problems. Through talk therapy, they provide tools and strategies for dealing with a variety of problems, from everyday stress to more serious mental health issues.

Psychiatrists

Psychiatrists are doctors who specialize in mental health. They can make a diagnosis, suggest therapy, and prescribe medications if necessary.

Safe Environment

Professional settings offer a confidential and non-judgmental space for people to express their concerns, fears, and problems. This environment promotes trust and open communication.

Early intervention

Seeking help early when symptoms or problems first appear can prevent more serious problems in the future. Early intervention often leads to more effective results.

Limit screen time

The digital revolution has brought countless benefits, but it also creates challenges. Excessive screen time, especially on social media, can have detrimental effects on mental well-being.

Digital Detox

Taking a periodic break from digital devices allows you to reset your mind. This allows you to take a break from the constant flow of information and notifications.

Scheduled breaks

Setting specific intervals throughout the day to step away from screens can reduce eye strain and mental fatigue. These breaks can be used for physical activity, meditation, or other non-digital activities.

Offline events

Engaging in non-screen activities, such as reading a physical book, crafting, or outdoor activities, can provide balance to digital consumption.

Curate digital content

Being selective about the content you consume online is critical. Unsubscribing from negative or triggering content and subscribing to uplifting, educational, or inspirational content can transform your digital experience.

Stay informed

Knowledge gives power. Gaining insight into your mental and emotional well-being, as well as the world around you, can lead to better decision-making and a deeper understanding of yourself and others.

Mental Health Education

Understanding the signs, symptoms and coping mechanisms for various mental health problems can be invaluable. This knowledge not only helps with self-awareness but also with supporting loved ones who may be experiencing difficulties.

Masterclasses and seminars

Attending a workshop, seminar, or webinar on mental health, mindfulness, or personal development can provide new ideas and tools for improving your well-being.

Stay updated

With the rapid development of psychology and neuroscience, discoveries and research are constantly emerging. Subscribing to reputable magazines, magazines or websites can keep you informed.

Positive environment

The environment, both physical and emotional, plays a key role in shaping a person's mental well-being. Surrounding yourself with positivity can promote optimism, resilience, and happiness.

Physical environment

An organized, clean, and aesthetically pleasing environment can boost your mood and productivity. Personalizing your space with items that bring joy, such as plants, art, or photographs, can make it more inviting and welcoming.

Social environment

Building and nurturing relationships with positive, supportive, and understanding people can create a protective network of trust and mutual respect. Avoiding or limiting interactions with negative or toxic people can also protect mental well-being.

Digital environment

In today's digital age, much of our environment is online. By creating a positive digital space, following uplifting content, limiting your exposure to negative news, and taking regular digital detoxes, you can have a significant impact on your mental health.

Do joyful things

Joy in its purest form can lift your spirits, rejuvenate your mind, and energize your body. Participating in activities that spark joy can be a transformative experience.

Hobbies

From painting to playing a musical instrument, from gardening to dancing, hobbies are personal interests that provide an escape from everyday stresses. They allow people to express themselves creatively and find purpose.

New experience

Exploring new activities or places can be exciting. Whether it's trying a new cuisine, taking a workshop, or traveling to a new place, these experiences can open up new perspectives and invigorate the soul.

Feeling of accomplishment

Completing a project, mastering a new skill, or achieving a personal goal brings a sense of pride and accomplishment. This feeling can improve self-esteem and overall well-being.

Social activity

Joyful activities are often more enriching when they are shared with others. Joining clubs, attending group activities, or simply sharing a hobby with a friend can enhance the joy experienced.

Mindfulness

In a world filled with distractions, being truly present in the moment is both a challenge and a necessity. Mindfulness is the practice of grounding oneself in the present, leading to increased awareness and calm.

Meditation

Meditation is a structured practice that promotes mindfulness. By focusing on your breath, a mantra, or simply observing your thoughts, meditation cultivates a deep sense of inner peace.

Deep breathing

Taking slow, intentional breaths can instantly ground a person in the present moment. Deep breathing exercises can be practiced anywhere and will instantly relieve you of stress and anxiety.

Observation without judgment

Mindfulness teaches the art of being an observer. Instead of reacting impulsively to thoughts or emotions, a person learns to observe them without judgment, realizing that they are temporary and do not define the person.

16

Physical Activity Types that should be part of your Daily Life

Different types of exercise have different advantages depending on individual goals, age, and health conditions. For those wanting to increase their strength or build muscle mass – weight training may be beneficial. Cardio exercises such as running or cycling can improve cardiovascular health and endurance, while activities like yoga and Pilates can help improve flexibility. For those wanting to lose weight, a combination of aerobic exercise, strength training, and a healthy diet are all important factors for success.

You should be mindful of your health and body strength conditions before you begin. It is advised to consult with your doctor about your plans for physical activity changes if you have health concerns, so you won't end up hurting yourself further.

When starting an exercise program, it is important to be realistic about what you can achieve and what kind of time frame you will set for yourself. Start slowly and build up gradually as your fitness level increases, ensuring that you warm up before any exercise session and cool down afterward. It is also important to set achievable goals so that you are more likely to stay motivated in the long run. Put your focus on short-term goals but have a vision for long-term health benefits.

Exercise is one of the major pillars in the foundation of our health. But with limited knowledge about which type of physical activity to add to our daily life, we tend to think that only one or two different types of activities are good enough. In reality, we should be mixing up four different ways of movement – aerobics, stretching, strength, and balance exercises.

Aerobic Exercise

If you are out of breath walking up the stairs, that is a clear indication that you need aerobic exercise to help with your heart, lungs, and endurance. It will help your muscles get sufficient blood flow and improve your heart and lung health. Aerobic exercise also lowers blood pressure, relaxes blood vessel walls, burns body fat, reduces inflammation, and raises good HDL cholesterol levels.

Adding walking, jogging, swimming, dancing, or any other aerobic exercises to your workout routine will help you reduce the risks of heart disease, stroke, breast cancer, and type 2 diabetes.

Stretching

When we talk about optimum health, we need to think long-term. Stretching is an exercise overlooked when we are younger but is a treasured addition to our regime. Aging causes loss of flexibility in tendons and muscles. Our muscles shorten and stop working properly. This can lead to body pains, cramps, muscle damage, strains, and joint pain.

Start stretching now, and your body will be thankful for years to come! As a beginner, start slowly and get deeper into your stretches as time passes and your body is more used to it. Aim to stretch at least 3-4 times per week.

Strength Training

We need to use our strength for daily, simple tasks – such as carrying grocery bags, lifting heavier objects around the house, or gardening. Having a body that feels good and can do necessary things without any struggles is important. That's what regular strength training helps with. Did you know that strengthening your muscles also helps with bone growth, assists weight control, lowers blood sugar, and reduces pain in joints?

You don't need fancy gym equipment for strength training. Bodyweight exercises are a good choice as well. Such as squats, lunges, or push-ups. But if you prefer to add some weights to your workouts, be mindful to get assistance from a trained professional who can guide you through every exercise. So your posture is correct, and you won't end up hurting yourself.

Balance Exercises

As we age, the systems that help us keep our balance start to break down – inner ear, vision, and muscles. So it is important to maintain good balance to avoid falls that can result in serious injuries. Training your balance can even prevent and reverse such breakdowns.

The best way to work on your balance is with tai chi, pilates, or yoga. Consult with a physical therapist to get the best balance exercises for your needs.

Exercise is one of the most important activities for maintaining good health. Different types of exercise can be tailored to different individuals to achieve specific goals. By making it part of your daily life, you can ensure that you are taking steps towards a healthier lifestyle. Consult with a doctor about which exercise routine fits best for your lifestyle and health conditions.

IV

Putting Knowledge into Action

17

Crafting Your Longevity Plan

There is a common belief that life expectancy depends largely on genetics. Many people repeat with satisfaction: "In my family, everyone lives to the age of ninety, we are long-lived," or: "I inherited my grandmother's genes, I am guaranteed to be in good health until I am one hundred!" However, it turns out that these genes play a much smaller role than originally thought.

Research clearly shows that environmental factors such as diet and healthy habits are key. This claim may also support the lifestyle that some celebrities lead. A prime example is certainly Jane Fonda, who, despite her 84 years of age, is still very physically active, something she has been encouraging women to do all over the world for almost 50 years. Many 30- or 40-year-olds can envy 70-year-old Sting's shape and sculpted body. According to the singer himself, in his case, it is due to yoga and avoiding meat in his diet. A similar approach is taken by the iconic wedding dress designer Vera Wang, who celebrated her 73rd birthday before the holidays and looks less than 30 (!) years old. Find out what habits you've observed among the stars will help you extend your life and, what's equally important, spend it in good shape.

Get enough sleep!

You have time for everything but sleep. You won't be able to go to bed before midnight, after all, you're addicted to the series, or you have a lot of work to do on an urgent project, a lot of ironing, or you're looking for your dream lamp on auction sites… But are these things more important? Uninterrupted sleep of adequate length, i.e. 7-8 hours a day, is crucial for the body. During this time, body cells and tissues are regenerated, and the body is cleansed of all unnecessary metabolic products, calming down inflammation, and also "resetting" the central nervous system. According to Healthline, according to the latest research, sleeping less than 5-7 hours a day is associated with a 12% higher risk of premature death. Too little sleep can also promote the development of many diseases: increasing the risk of diabetes, heart disease, and depression.

Become a flexitarian

You've heard it ad nauseam, but it's time to say it again. An appropriate diet based on vegetables, fruits, grains, nuts, and healthy vegetable oils is the key to maintaining health, which, of course, also affects life expectancy. Highly processed dishes and excess sugar should be excluded from the daily menu, and the amount of meat eaten should be minimized (it is best to eat it once or twice a week), as flexitarians do. When thinking about what you will cook, follow the example of the Mediterranean diet, which has been considered the healthiest in the world. Tomatoes, zucchini, eggplants, garlic, fresh fish, and olive oil should dominate your plate. It is also important not to overeat. In Japan, the largest number of centenarians live on the island of Okinawa. When scientists looked at their lifestyle and diet, it turned out that they ate small portions of low-calorie dishes - a total of about 1,900 kcal per day, and their BMI was 18-22. They have no weight fluctuations or obesity problems.

Eliminate cigarette smoke from your life

If you smoke cigarettes yourself or someone around you, you must know that the health consequences of inhaling cigarette smoke are disastrous for your health. Why? There are thousands of chemicals in cigarette smoke. Many of them are highly toxic or even carcinogenic. We are talking about tar substances, including radioactive polonium, nickel, hydrogen cyanide, ammonia, DDT (an ingredient of rodent poisons), and high concentrations of carbon monoxide. Smoking cigarettes damages the lungs and heart and increases the risk of stroke. The list of diseases seems endless. Therefore, if you plan to live a long life, you must quit cigarettes.

If you have tried to do this many times without success, consider plan B. You can start with nicotine replacement therapy (nicotine products such as gum or patches). If they do not help, use pharmaceuticals that suppress nicotine cravings, prescribed by a doctor. During the transitional period, a tobacco heater or e-cigarette may also be an alternative. Some of such products have already been thoroughly medically tested. For example, scientists from the National Institute of Public Health and the Environment in the Netherlands (RIVM) in a toxicological study estimated that a smoker using tobacco heated in an IQOS device exposes his body to 8 main carcinogenic compounds up to 25 times less than smoking cigarettes.

Researchers from RIVM also found that smokers who replace cigarettes with such a device have a much lower risk of premature death from cancer than cigarette smokers. Remember, however, that the most important goal should always be to break the addiction.

Do preventive tests

Your body needs an annual check-up to make sure nothing bad is happening. Most of us visit the dentist once a year to check the condition of our teeth, and perform cytology and breast ultrasound (you do them, right?!?), but the list of annual preventive examinations is also worth including blood count, blood glucose level, and blood pressure check. , and once every three years, a lipid profile.

Older people have too high cholesterol, glucose levels, or blood pressure problems. It may suddenly turn out that your sleep problems are caused by too high blood pressure, and the weakness and lack of energy to act are the result of too few red blood cells. Monitoring your health will reduce your risk of atherosclerosis, heart attack, stroke, or diabetes in the future. Each of these civilization's diseases reduces the quality of life and shortens its length.

Find time for physical activity and meeting friends

Specialists recommend spending 150 minutes a week on physical activity because this amount of exercise and sport helps keep the body in good condition. Does that seem like a lot to you? Not at all. This means that you should spend an average of 25 minutes a day exercising. It doesn't have to be heavy interval training every day. All you need is a quick walk, climbing the stairs to the fourth floor, cycling, jogging, yoga, or exercises done at home, such as squats, bends, swings, and running in place. A sedentary lifestyle is unnatural for humans, although many people function this way. If you want to be fit and healthy in retirement, you must get up from the couch as often as possible, since you can't get away from your desk at work.

Another important activity that affects life expectancy is... social activity. As the Human Population Laboratory's nine-year study of a random sample of 6,928 adults in Alameda County, California shows, loneliness and a lack of lasting social connections contribute to higher mortality rates. Scientists who examined the "blue zones", i.e. those places in the world with the highest average life expectancy, reached similar conclusions. These include the already mentioned Japanese Okinawa, as well as Sardinia in Italy, Greek Ikaria, the Hunza Valley in the Himalayas, and villages in the Caucasus. Each of these places differs in culture, customs, and diet, but what they have in common is that people live there in very close family and neighborly relationships.

Living a long life when you are young seems obvious. However, what also matters is its quality. Of course, you have no direct influence on many matters. You cannot single-handedly change carbon dioxide emissions into the atmosphere or stop the melting of glaciers. But you can influence what you eat, whether you take care of your relationships with friends, and whether you poison your body with cigarettes. If you want to live long and well, start doing it today!

18

Make a life plan

Our lives are constantly changing. When you feel like you're just going with the flow, or you're questioning your priorities, creating a life plan can help change your situation. With a life plan, you can organize your life despite changes. In this chapter, you will learn how to create your life plan.

Prioritization

Think about what your current role is

Every day we play different roles. Depending on our actions, during the day we can be "daughter", "artist", "student", "girlfriend", "cheese lover", etc. Write your list on a piece of paper. Try to place these roles in the correct order, paying attention to their priority.

Here are some examples of other roles like Chef, Dog Walker, Brother, Photographer, Chef, Mentor, Traveler, Grandson, Thinker, etc.

Think about the role you would like to play in the future

Some, if not all, of the roles you currently have in your life you will likely want to continue to play in the future, such as continuing to be a "mother" or an "artist." However, these roles are just names, and every person would want someone to use them to describe them at the end of their lives. Think about the negative roles you currently play - perhaps roles that you would like to cross off your list as you plan for your future.

To create your list, think about what you would like to do in the future. Do you want to travel but have never done it before? If so, add the role of "traveler" to your future list.

Think about your motives

Why do you want to play these roles in the future? To create a life plan, you need to properly prioritize your life. To do this, think about the roles you want to continue playing, as well as the ones you want to add in the future. Think about why you want to play a certain role. Maybe you want to become a "father", then among your future goals write down your desire to have children with your partner, and give the child life.

A simple way to figure out the reasons for your ambitions is this: imagine your funeral (even though it's painful, it needs to be done, it helps!) Who will attend it? What would you like people to say about you? Perhaps you would like to hear the most important words, such as that you were an amazing mother or made an effort to help thousands of homeless animals.

Write down your priorities

Once you understand your motivations, write them down. Making a list will help you stay organized as you begin to follow your plan.

For example, the list might include: I am a 'sister' because I always want to be a support for my brother; I want to be a "writer" because I can write down the story of my grandparents, etc.

Think about your physical and emotional needs

What does it take to become who you want to be? For example, if you want to become an "Everest climber", you must be physically fit and eat right. If you want to be a "friend", your emotional needs will be met if you surround yourself with loving people.

Setting Goals

Think about what goals you want to achieve throughout your life

Use your roles, priorities, and needs and you will be able to understand what you want in your life. Think about this list in terms of things you want to get done before you die. Remember that these should be goals that you want to achieve and not goals that others encourage you to achieve. If you need more help, try categorizing your goals. Some examples of categories:

Career/Vocation; Society (family and friends); Finance, health, travel Knowledge / Intelligence and Spirituality.

Example goal (according to category): become a famous architect; get married and have two children; earn enough money to give a good education to your children; stay in good shape; visit all continents; obtain a master's degree in architecture; visit the Buddhist temple Borobudur.

Write down specific goals with specific dates

Once you have set a goal that you want to achieve in your life, such as getting a degree, write it down along with the date by which you want to achieve your goal. Here are some goals that are less vague than those listed in the previous step:

- Lose 5kg by June 2023.
- Be accepted into the Master's program in Architecture by April 2025.
- Travel to Indonesia to visit Borobudur Temple in 2026.

Think about how you will achieve your goals

To do this, you need to evaluate where you are right now. The steps you need to take will depend on what you are currently doing. For example, to obtain a master's degree in architecture.

From now until April 2015, you will need to: A. Study architecture programs. B. Complete the required application. B. Complete the rest of the application and submit it to the appropriate authorities. D. Wait for an answer. Select the program you would like to study. E. Sign up!

Planning

Write down what actions you need to take to achieve each goal

You can do this in any format - by hand, type a Word document, draw on a large sheet of paper, etc. Whatever format you use, write down what actions you will need to take to achieve each of your goals in chronological order. Congratulations - you've just created your life plan.

Now is the time to study the details of each step - the name of specific master's programs. Or, if one of your goals is to simply be happy, write down in detail what will make you happiest in this life.

Check your life plan.

Life changes and so do we. The goals and priorities we had at 15 will likely be different from the goals we will have at 25 or 45. It is important to periodically review your life plan to check whether you are following it in your life, this will allow you to lead a happy and satisfied life.

When checking your life plan, also evaluate your progress. Be sure to track your achievements.

Adjust your life plan

When you see that your priorities and goals have changed, rewrite the part of your life plan that needs changing. Think about what has changed, what is more important to you now, and what you will do to achieve the new goal. Rewrite your life plan to suit your circumstances.

Don't limit yourself to a certain number of goals. Add goals as they become a priority in your life, and remove from the list those that are not so important to you.

Advise

Constantly review and adjust your plan. Your life will constantly change and so will your plan.

Don't be too hard on yourself if you can't achieve the goal by the date you set make adjustments to the plan and continue to follow it further.

19

Strategies for turning obstacles into opportunities

There is an old story about a king whose subjects became too soft and inactive. Disappointed with this state of affairs, he decided to teach them a lesson. His plan was simple: place a large boulder in the middle of the main road and block the entrance to the city. After which he hid nearby and watched. What will the residents do? Maybe they can team up to remove the boulder? Or will they become discouraged and give up?

With growing disappointment, the king watched as his subjects approached the boulder, turned around, and walked away. At best, one of them tried to move the stone alone, but then also left. Many openly complained or scolded the king, but no one could or wanted to do anything about it.

A few days later, a peasant passed along the road. He didn't turn around. Instead, he harnessed his horse and tried to move the boulder. Then he came up with an idea: he went into the nearby forest to find something he could use as leverage. Finally, he returned with a large branch, from which he made a lever and used it to move the boulder out of the way.

Under the rock was a purse of gold coins and a note from the king that said: "An obstacle in the path becomes part of the path. Never forget that every obstacle holds an opportunity."

Here are nine strategies to help you overcome obstacles along the way.

Change Your Perspective

By controlling our emotions, we learn to understand that an event and a reaction to an event are completely different things. An event is objective, but the reaction to it can be subjective.

Any obstacle, any problem can be turned into an opportunity if you calm down your emotions and take a closer look. Perception is what is very important. It guides our thoughts, our words, our actions, and our deeds. If you have the right perception, then everything else will work itself out.

Turn the Obstacle on its Head

Laura Ingalls Wilder believed:
"There is good in everything, you just have to look patiently
."

Events that we initially perceive as negative contain positive, overt benefits. You just need to recognize it. Suppose you typed text for a long time without saving it, a crash occurred and everything was deleted. Of course, time cannot be returned. But now you can write a second time - better and faster because you are already prepared.

Always Stay Moving

Theodore Roosevelt said:

> "We can all either wear out or rust. My choice is to wear myself out."

Usually, the winners are those who attack their problems first and prevent them. Such people have more energy not because their body is designed this way, but because they are accustomed to this rhythm.

Courage is simply the ability to take action. Start by saying yes to new challenges and start moving without stopping. Wake up in the morning and immediately get down to business: no need to laze in bed or drink coffee for half an hour. This will only waste your time doing nothing.

Obstacles appear more daunting to us when we stop to take a closer look at them.

Fail Cheaply

Wendell Phillips:

> "What is defeat? Nothing but a lesson. Nothing but the first steps towards something better."

Engineers like to joke: a bug is a feature. There's nothing wrong with being wrong. Every time something bad happens, new opportunitie open up and problems become apparent.

When failure occurs, ask yourself: why did it happen? This helps to find alternative ways to solve the problem. Failure puts us in a corner and, with our backs against the wall, we tend to do great things.

Follow the Plan

In the chaos of life, a plan creates a route for us. After every problem or failure, take a break and catch your breath. Something went wrong. This means we need to adjust the plan and solve the problem.

Some people don't follow a plan when chaos and destruction set in. But in vain: even a bad plan is better than its complete absence.

What works is right

Deng Xiaoping was pragmatic:

> "I don't care whether the cat is black or white as long as it catches mice."

We spend a lot of time thinking about how things should be. But what difference does it make in how things should be if reality is reality? Start thinking like a radical pragmatist: don't change the world right now. But be ambitious enough to get what you need now.

Use Obstacles Against Themselves

Plutarch believed:

> "Wise people know how to use even their enemies correctly."

Sometimes you can overcome obstacles by using them to your advantage rather than by fighting them. Thus, a castle may seem like a formidable fortress. But it can be turned into a prison for the people inhabiting it if surrounded.

Instead of starting to fight obstacles, think about how to force them to defeat themselves.

Take Your Chance

Edwin Chapin is sure:

> "The best people are not those who wait for a chance, but those who take advantage of them."

Ordinary people avoid difficult situations and troubles. What great people do is the opposite of such actions. They never lose the opportunity to turn a personal tragedy or crisis to their advantage.

At certain times we face great challenges. And we must see that all these "problems" open up opportunities for solutions that we have been waiting for a long time.

Focus on something bigger than yourself

Leroy Percy believed:

> "Man's task is to make the world a better place to live in and to care for his soul."

When we are faced with some impossible task, one of the best ways to create an opportunity is to ask ourselves the question: "If I can't solve it for myself, how can I solve it for other people?" You'll be amazed at how many solutions you can find if you start thinking about something bigger.

20

10 Steps to Achieve Your Goals

To achieve success in any endeavor, you need a system of consistent actions. Many people believe that it is enough to just define a goal and go towards it, but everything is not so simple. If the goal is long-term, then you risk encountering obstacles that you may not have enough motivation or inspiration to overcome. And only a systematic approach will help you out.

Reaching a goal is like a long, grueling race. Someone may start running fast and after a short period, they will fall exhausted. And someone will distribute them over the entire distance and cross the finish line. We bring to your attention a system of 10 steps that will help ensure that you do not run out of steam immediately after the start.

Choose a goal that motivates and inspires you

You shouldn't set such a banal goal as learning English. That is, of course, there may be such a goal, but you must approach the formulation of the task itself differently. For example: learning to speak fluently without feeling awkward in conversations with native speakers, or learning to read and understand books in English.

One of the keys to successfully achieving a goal (besides discipline) is motivation. When you set it, make sure it is important to you and aligns with your values. That is, the goal must have clearly defined benefits. It also needs to be relevant to the overall picture of your life. When you set it up, make sure you're very committed to achieving it by doing the following:

1. Ask yourself if you are putting it because you want to achieve something or because it is fashionable and popular. Are your interests and needs taken into account? After all, you will have to go to the goal for a long time, so you need to make sure that you need it.
2. Ask yourself: "On a scale of 1 to 10, how much do I need this?"
3. Write down all the benefits you expect to receive if you achieve your goal.
4. Ask yourself, "How does this goal fit into the big picture of my life?"

Move to step two when you are confident that you are motivated enough to achieve this goal.

Make it specific

You've probably heard it a million times: vague goals produce vague results. If you want positive, clear results, your goals must be specific. Let's say you want to read 30 classic fiction books over the next year. To do this you need:

1. Write down the titles of all the works you want to read. Spend

enough time compiling a list of books that interest you.

2. Determine whether they will be in electronic or paper format.
3. Decide how much time you will spend reading.

Look at your goal and ask yourself, "How can I make it more specific?" Then ask again, "How can I make it even more specific?" In our case, the answer will be: "Read one book from the list every week."

Set a deadline

Deadlines are one of the best motivators in life. They are vital to achieving your goal. Whatever goal you choose, make sure there is a deadline.

Set milestones

The main stage is the transition from one phase to another. When a goal is too far away, milestones act as signposts to track your progress and make sure you're on the right track. They also allow you to see where there is a reason to rejoice and celebrate, which is also important for the motivation and continuation of the movement.

Find out what the main steps are on the way to your goal. This is important for the next step.

Reward yourself

Rewards are a great incentive to work towards your goals. Ideally, however, the process of achieving a goal will be a reward in itself. But even if you love to read, sometimes reading will be very difficult.

Rewards can be quite symbolic and cost you pennies. Enjoy the process, but don't forget about the little well-deserved joys of life.

Break the path to your goal into separate steps

One of the main reasons people put off their goals is because they don't know how to take action. Therefore, you must know what to do. That is, break it down into small steps.

Any goal can be broken down into smaller ones. For example:

1. If your goal is to write a novel, then the goal will be a certain number of pages or chapters written.
2. If the goal is to learn a foreign language, then the goal will be to complete 3 lessons in a week.

Write down these small step goals.

Plan it out

Once you know exactly what you'll be doing each day, it's time to start planning.

Make sure that there are no other things planned and that you will not be distracted by anyone or anything. Of course, this includes muting your cell phone.

Track your progress

There is research that shows that tracking your progress toward goals improves your well-being and happiness. By evaluating your results, you will ensure that you are going in the right direction. All this will ultimately give even more motivation.

When you fall, get up

In pursuit of a goal, you will fall more than once (that's why we say "when" and not "if"). It is important to be mentally prepared for the fact that there will be defeats.

You may also fall behind your plan for various reasons: illness, other commitments, or difficult circumstances. Don't give up - get back to work as soon as you can. Don't let failure distract you from your goal.

Find a way to hold yourself accountable to your goal

You need to commit to achieving your goal, otherwise it will be very easy to give up on it when times get tough (and they will). If possible, work on your goal with other people. For example, write a novel together. It may be chaotic, but this way it will be easier to motivate each other.

21

Achievement motivation

Motivation is the driving force behind human actions. Individual needs, ambitions, and desires have a strong influence on the direction of our behavior. We satisfy our needs in different ways and strive for success for different reasons, both personal and general. There are various forms of motivation such as extrinsic, intrinsic, physiological, and achievement.

Achievement motivation can be defined as the need for improvement with the basis for the triumph of all our aspirations in life. Goals influence how we perform tasks and reflect urges to demonstrate our skills. These basic physiological aspects influence natural human behavior in various conditions.

Motivation can range from biological needs to satisfying creative desires or achieving success in competitive endeavors. That's why it's so important because it affects life every day. All our behavior, actions, thoughts, and beliefs are influenced by the internal desire for success, the desire to feel the pleasant weight of a laurel wreath on our heads.

History and Research

The study of achievement motivation has a long and distinguished history. Scientists have focused on this question since the dawn of psychology as a scientific discipline—when William James made suggestions about how skill propensity relates to self-esteem.

Currently, this topic is an area of active research, especially in the fields of educational psychology, sport and exercise psychology, industrial psychology, and social psychology of personality and development. Research is conducted both in experimental laboratories (where variables are typically used) and in real-world settings such as classrooms, workplaces, or sports fields.

The task is to explain and predict any behavior associated in one way or another with the ability principle. Examples of goal strivings are ubiquitous in life and present in many different situations. For example, a gardener striving to grow the perfect orchid, a teenager who wants to become a good communicator, or an elderly person concerned about the gradual loss of his abilities.

Over time, numerous steps have been taken in attempts to understand what achievement motivation is. Among them, it is worth highlighting:

1. The desire for success. The level of efficiency we want or don't want to achieve. Research by Kurt Lewin and Ferdinand Hoppe
2. Needs and motives. General, emotional predisposition to success and failure. Research by David McClelland and John Atkinson
3. Anxiety testing. Anxiety and nervousness a possible influences on the quality of work. Research by Charles Spielberger and Martin

Covington

4. Functionality in achieving goals. Ideas about the reasons for positive and negative results. Research by Bernard Weiner and Heinz Heckhausen

5. Goals to achieve. Ideas about the successes or failures that people strive to achieve or avoid. Research by Carol Dweck and John Nichols

6. Implicit theories of ability. Exploring the nature of competence and ability. Research by Carol Dweck and Robert Sternberg

7. Presumed knowledge. Understanding what can and cannot be achieved. Research by Albert Bandura and Susan Harter.

8. Appreciating the importance of success or avoiding failure. Research by Jacqueline Eccles, Judy Harakiewicz

Many scholars have focused on one of the above factors in their work, while others have sought to integrate two or more of these dimensions into an overall conceptual framework.

McClelland's study of need

Achievement theory (or need for achievement) was primarily promoted by American psychologist David McClelland. He spent much of his life developing the idea that three key needs are acquired through learning or experience. They cannot be learned at some seminars, but you can still learn them if you practice for several months or a year. What are these three needs:

1. Need for achievement. Selecting situations where success depends on performance

2. The need to belong. Essentially, being close to someone. Such a person enjoys mutual friendship with others

3. Need for strength. Those who have this need have a great need to control events and things or influence others

Five Characteristics of a High Need for Achievement

Going for a personal record

Edmund Hilary, who, together with his guide, Nepalese Sherpa Tenzing Norgay, became the first person to climb Everest, the highest mountain peak on earth. Few of us are truly capable of doing this, but those who do have an undeniable drive to succeed. And the point is not to increase financial earnings. It's about achieving a goal, and then an even more difficult goal, in the pursuit of perfection, without becoming an obsessive perfectionist.

Setting moderate goals, understanding and calculating possible risks

This is not calculating probabilities using cold mathematics. It's a compromise between easy and too hard. Let's imagine that you are going to throw a ring on a stick. You can choose how far or how close you want to stand from this ring. Some people will stand very close to success every time. Others will risk standing too far, so they only manage to throw the hoop on rare occasions, and mostly because they get lucky. And someone, to achieve satisfaction, will choose the distance at which he will use exactly the skill necessary to succeed. With the condition that there will be no problems, but it will not be too easy.

Personal responsibility in finding solutions to problems

Such a person enjoys the feeling of his readiness to solve difficult situations. In some cases, he does this completely voluntarily.

Striving for unique achievements, tirelessness, and innovation

At first glance, it may seem that like these people, there is an element of inconsistency and non-conformism. They are not good candidates for a bank job where transactions must be done the same day after day, without change. Do you remember the name of the person who served you the last time you visited the bank?

For example, Steve Jobs was a bit of a nonconformist in his early years. The story goes that he was able to get his first job simply by asking the person who could hire him. At the same time, he did not cut his hair and did not bother to wear shoes to the meeting. He simply found someone who could hire him and asked to get himself a job.

How different is this from our usual understanding of an interview, where we must fully adhere to the dress code and have a resume that Superman would envy?

Of course, this inconsistency is both a blessing and a curse for a standardized organization with defined and well-organized processes. Therefore, each employee with the same job title should have approximately the same behavior. And a person with a high need and desire to innovate should conform to the rules or leave.

Search for negative feedback

There is an expression - a true friend is the one who tells you about your weaknesses and does not praise you for your strengths. The average person is afraid of negative reviews. We don't want to hear about our mistakes, failures, and what we could have done better.

People who have the above characteristics are indeed special to some extent. They view negative rather than positive feedback as more valuable. The reason is the desire to make oneself more perfect. And to understand how to achieve this, you need to know what to improve or upgrade.

www.ingramcontent.com/pod-product-compliance
Lightning Source LLC
Chambersburg PA
CBHW061638250726

48659CB00004B/1285